Late Preterm Infants

Shahirose Sadrudin Premji
Editor

Late Preterm Infants

A Guide for Nurses, Midwives, Clinicians and Allied Health Professionals

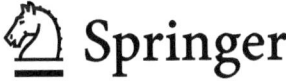 Springer

Editor
Shahirose Sadrudin Premji
School of Nursing, Faculty of Health
York University
Toronto
ON
Canada

With illustrations by Bronwyn AC Martin

ISBN 978-3-319-94351-0   ISBN 978-3-319-94352-7   (eBook)
https://doi.org/10.1007/978-3-319-94352-7

Library of Congress Control Number: 2018957082

This Springer imprint is published by the registered company Springer Nature Switzerland AG
The registered company address is: Gewerbestrasse 11, 6330 Cham, Switzerland

Preface

Although late preterm infants (born between $34^{0/7}$ and $36^{6/7}$ weeks' gestational age) account for a large proportion (75%) of preterm infants, they have received little attention with respect to developing best practices to care for them. Bernie Schrage is a public health nurse who has been instrumental in my journey in learning about the unique characteristics of late preterm infants and the trials and tribulations their mothers and fathers experience when caring for them in the early days following discharge. Her passion fueled and continues to fuel the desire to educate others about the very special needs of late preterm infants and the importance of educating and supporting mothers and father to enhance their self-efficacy and self-confidence in caring for their very special babies.

Toronto, ON, Canada   Shahirose Sadrudin Premji

Acknowledgement

Every wish has a little miracle waiting to be realized!
Shahirose Sadrudin Premji

There were many sparks that ignited the wish to write this book.

My mother who gave birth to my sister and me earlier than anticipated at about 32 weeks' of gestation (moderate preterm) and 36 weeks' of gestation (late preterm), respectively. We were born in Dar-es-Salaam, Tanzania a low- and middle-income country with limited resources to care for preterm infants, especially like my sister who was 2 pounds and 8 ounces. My sister was fed with cotton soaked in milk that was then pressed at her lips to release the milk one drop at a time! The doctors ordered a "special dropper" from Nairobi, Kenya to feed her. She remained in the hospital for 1 month. I was lucky and come home much earlier but my mother had "complications" so needed to stay in hospital much longer. The book is an expression of gratitude to my mother for giving us birth, nurturing us, and sacrificing so much to ensure we have a good life!

My father whose love, determination, and sacrifices brought us to Canada so we could access the best knowledge and have a future. My parents have instilled in us to give the gift of knowledge to others. The book is a gift!

My sister and brother-in-law who have been my pillars of strength, as well have encouraged and supported my international work. I will be forever grateful for their unconditional love, kindness, generosity, and care given to my parents. I am so blessed to have you in my life! Shukhar!

The nurses, midwives, and doctors in Tanzania who innovated to care for my sister and me and ensure we survived and went home!

All mothers, fathers, late preterm infants, and health care providers who have touched my life and helped me appreciate how special late preterm infants are including all those who care for them. In essence, it is their story(ies) that shape our knowledge and best practices in caring for late preterm infants and their families.

All the authors who embraced the opportunity to write the chapters with enthusiasm and have so willingly shared their time, knowledge, and experience in writing the chapter(s). Their dedication to the book, the late preterm infants and their families, and commitment to improving the care and outcomes of late preterm infants and their families is appreciated more than words can express.

The illustrator Bronwyn Martin, whose talents far surpass her young age. A gifted young artist who has amazed me!!

All my family and friends who have believed in me, who have helped me be strong in the face of adversity and who celebrated me no matter what. Thank you!

The book is an expression of gratitude to all the wonderful people who have touched my life and helped me appreciate that every person has potential and nothing is impossible. May your wish – the potential and the possibilities – be realized!

Contents

Contributors

Gisela Becker, RM, MA Department of Health and Community Services, Government of Newfoundland and Labrador, St. John's, NL, Canada

Katherine Bright, RN, BSc, BN, MN, PhD(C) Faculty of Nursing, University of Calgary, Calgary, AB, Canada

Women's Mental Health Clinic, Alberta Health Services, Calgary, AB, Canada

Dianne Creighton, PhD Neonatal Follow-Up Clinic, Alberta Children's Hospital, Calgary, AB, Canada

Department of Paediatrics, Cumming School of Medicine, University of Calgary, Calgary, AB, Canada

Genevieve Currie, RN, MN School of Nursing and Midwifery, Mount Royal University, Calgary, AB, Canada

Aliyah Dosani, RN, BN, MPH, PhD School of Nursing and Midwifery, Mount Royal University, Calgary, AB, Canada

Department of Community Health Sciences, Cumming School of Medicine, University of Calgary, Calgary, AB, Canada

Susan Kau, BSN, RNC-NIC Caring for Hawai'i Neonates, Honolulu, HI, USA

Council of International Neonatal Nurses, Inc. (COINN), Yardley, PA, USA

Carole Kenner, RN, PhD, FAAN, FNAP, ANEF School of Nursing and Health and Exercise Science, The College of New Jersey, New York, NY, USA

Council of International Neonatal Nurses, Inc. (COINN), Yardley, PA, USA

Mary R. Landsiedel, BN, BMid, MMid Bachelor of Midwifery Program, School of Nursing and Midwifery, Mount Royal University, Calgary, AB, Canada

Karen Lasby, RN, BScN, MN, CNeoN(C) Neonatal Transition Team, Postpartum Services, Calgary, AB, Canada

Abhay K. Lodha, MBBS, MD, DM, MSC Department of Paediatrics, Cumming School of Medicine, University of Calgary, Calgary, AB, Canada

Department of Community Health Sciences, Cumming School of Medicine, University of Calgary, Calgary, AB, Canada

Department of Paeditrics, Foothills Medical Center C211, Alberta Health Services, Calgary, AB, Canada

Jennifer Marandola, RN, BScN, MN, IBCLC, PNC(C) Volet Jeunesse/Santé-Publique, Centre Intégré Universitaire de Santé et de Services Sociaux de l'Ouest-de-l'île-de-Montréal, Montréal, QC, Canada

Lenora Marcellus, RN, BSN, MN, PhD School of Nursing, University of Victoria, Victoria, BC, Canada

Allison C. Munn, RN, PhD Department of Nursing, Francis Marion University, Florence, SC, USA

Gianella Santos Pana Birth Doula, Chavah Childbirth Services Inc., Calgary, AB, Canada

Faculty of Nursing, University of Calgary, Calgary, AB, Canada

Shahirose Sadrudin Premji, RN, BSc, BScN, MScN, PhD, FAAN School of Nursing, Faculty of Health, York University, Toronto, ON, Canada

Janet M. Rankin, RN PhD Faculty of Nursing, University of Calgary, Calgary, AB, Canada

Catherine Ringham, RN BSN PhD CNeoN(C) Faculty of Nursing, University of Calgary, Calgary, AB, Canada

Sarah N. Taylor, MD Department of Pediatrics, Medical University of South Carolina, Charleston, SC, USA

Who Is the Late Preterm Infant and What Problems Can Arise for This Population

Shahirose Sadrudin Premji and Susan Kau

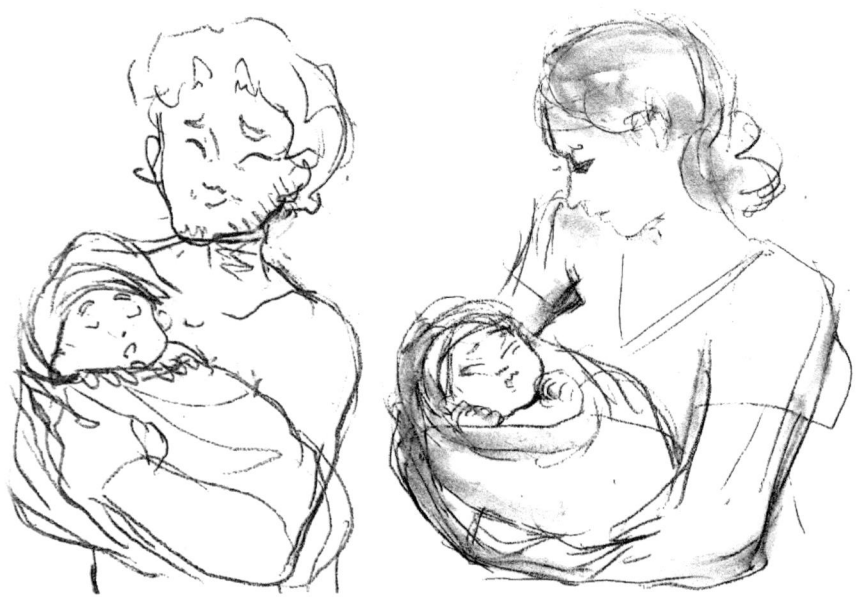

S. S. Premji (✉)
School of Nursing, Faculty of Health, York University, Toronto, ON, Canada
e-mail: premjis@yorku.ca

S. Kau
Caring for Hawai'i Neonates, Honolulu, HI, USA

Council of International Neonatal Nurses, Inc. (COINN), Yardley, PA, USA

The inspiration and guiding light for this chapter comes from insight learned from caring for late preterm infants William and Andrew K. (twins), Asher K., and Tyler N.—who in their own little ways invited curiosity and imparted knowledge to help us understand their developmental trajectories and potential.

We are a unique population—medical and textbooks categorize us as the 34 0/7–36 6/7 weekers or late preterm infants (LPIs). Other terms used to describe us such as near term or almost term do not address important concepts that our brain, lungs, and other systems still have at least 6 weeks to grow, and this time is critical to our growth and development [1]. We will share with you how to best care for our needs so that you don't treat us like term babies [2]. In some NICUs, we outnumber the patient population of micropremies, term, and post-term infants [3]. The late pre-term infants are the new "baby boomers."

How we adjust to life outside mom's belly (i.e., womb or uterus) is affected by how health-care providers care for our mothers when they are in labor and when they deliver us. Maternal management and its impacts on LPI morbidities such as hypoglycemia, glucose metabolism, and hyperinsulinism are discussed in Chap. 2. Our clinical problems may include some or all of the following: respiratory distress, apnea, bradycardia, and desaturations also known as A/B/Ds, temperature instabil-ity, hypoglycemia, and hyperbilirubinemia, as well as being "problematic" in breast- and bottle-feeding [2, 4].

Even though we have many potential problems, my mom has a one in four chance of developing anxiety and/or depression during pregnancy [5, 6]. Other factors such as her labor and delivery experience, how well she is doing during and after deliv-ery, and worrying about me possibly coming out earlier may play a role in why I am a LPI [7, 8]. My brain function is impacted by my mom's emotional well-being. So please read Chap. 3 which explains how care providers can start to identify risk fac-tors regarding her emotional health early on so that they can take care of her so she can take care of me [9, 10].

On another note, please don't forget about my dad—this is in Chap. 4. The lack of knowledge about me and my problems challenges him [11]. My unexpected early delivery/birth places him in a lot of stress as well. He oftentimes needs to make decisions about me as well as support my mom as she recovers from giving birth to me. He also has to update all of the rest of the family and friends about me and my mom. So please don't forget to communicate with him with concise and consistent information. It will be the key to enhancing my parent-infant relationship—a once-in-a-lifetime experience!!

My nurses in the neonatal intensive care unit are an amazing breed!! They are our "voices" and advocates, and their #1 priority is me, my comfort, safety, and enhanc-ing the patient experience for me and my family. Research tells us they experience many challenges in practicing their passion; read Chap. 5. They watch me "out the corners of their eyes," but I do need their full attention. It is not their fault though as they are often asked to do more with less. The nurses are trying so hard to be respon-sive to my special needs, but "boy do they have a ton of policies to follow." The technology can be tricky and again with those policies! Chapter 5 helps us under-stand how hard the nurses try to make me a priority in the care.

We offer challenges like no other in terms of timing of our discharge. Although some of us are larger than someone else with our same gestation, we are not all the same!! We are all individuals with different names and personalities. Just remember "we call the shots!!" It is not uncommon for us to try the "patience" of our caregivers (medical doctors, nurses, midwives, medical doctors physical therapists, occupational therapists, speech therapists, and especially our parents who want us home). During medical rounds, please call us by our first names—it makes us feel special.

1.1 Here Are Some of the Challenges We Offer in the Hospital

Respiratory issues—some of us need assistance after birth to breathe. New words for our parents and in our own vocabulary include oxygen, ventilator, nasal intermittent positive pressure ventilation (NIPPV), continuous positive airway pressure (CPAP), high-flow nasal cannula (HFNC), low-flow nasal cannula (LFNC), surfactant, apnea, desaturations, pulse oximetry, and caffeine to name a few. We need you to look for signs that we are working hard with our breathing—breathing too fast (more than 60 breaths per minute) with shallow breaths (tachypnea), the opening of the nose widen (nasal flaring), the skin and muscle between and around the chest pull sharply (retractions), and noise when we breathe out (grunting)—and act quickly; otherwise, we may stop breathing altogether [12].

Apnea, bradycardia, and desaturations or A/B/Ds—we alert our nurses and parents with our A/B/Ds by setting off our alarms which keeps my nurses on their toes [13]. Our control of breathing, heart rate, and sleep state is not fully developed, but we get better with time (i.e., postnatal age). We do have a higher rate of sudden infant death syndrome (also known as cot or crib death which is unexplained in early infancy that is prior to 1 year of age) compared to babies that are born full-term [13].

Hypoglycemia—our glucose levels fall after birth and can remain low for a few hours, while we learn to make our own glucose, but we also have trouble maintaining the right level of sugar in our blood [14]. One request we have is that you watch us closely, especially if our mothers also had sugar problems, so that you protect our brain [14]—read more about this in Chap. 2. In the "golden hour," the first hour after birth, let my mother provide skin-to-skin or kangaroo care—you can dry me, and leave me undressed on my mother's naked chest, and cover me with a blanket or towel [15]. Please don't separate me from my mother—unless I'm doing something silly like not breathing—and let her feed me every 2–3 hours, and monitor my blood sugars initially until they remain stable [14].

Temperature instability—we are especially vulnerable to hypothermia which can lead to a whole cascade of problems for us including increase oxygen consumption which can lead to hypoxia, increase glucose utilization, and depletion of glycogen stores which can lead to hypoglycemia [16]. More new words to learn here is incubator (isolette), servocontrol skin probe (ISC) vs neutral thermal environment (NTE) mode, and bassinet to crib. Since we are not quite term, we lack enough brown fat (substance that is accumulated in increasing amounts as the infant advances through gestation) [16]. Please help us conserve our body heat by helping maintain a normal body temperature [16]—another benefit of kangaroo care here. The next step for us is "wean to crib." This is a period of time when we are trending adequate weight gain with less to no support from our incubators. We now graduate, so we can wear clothes, be swaddled, and placed in a bassinet. One step closer to home. Yeah!!

Please share the benefits of kangaroo care with my parents and encourage my mom and dad to do kangaroo care when they are visiting us. We appreciate "quiet times" as well as having our cares and exams clustered. If you notice my skin has spots or blotches of red and white—I am *stressed*!! One request we have is to please help us to rest and grow by positioning us comfortably using developmental support aids and guidelines.

1.2   Here Are Some of the Challenges That May Be Ongoing During Our Transition Home

We have a higher risk of readmission rates due to hyperbilirubinemia, feeding difficulties, and respiratory issues like bronchitis, pneumonia, and respiratory syncytial virus (RSV) in particular [17–19]. Chapter 7 explains why I'm a frequent flyer to the hospital in the first year of life. There are lots of good strategies for you to learn and share with my parents. Hyperbilirubinemia—the key here is to educate my family (especially first-time mothers) on how to evaluate feedings and what signs to look for to detect dehydration and jaundice. Feeding issues—bottle-feeding and breastfeeding seem to be the biggest hurdle for us and require two chapters!! Chapter 8 explains why it is so hard to feed me and gives health-care providers and my mother some strategies to consider. Please don't call us "wimps" and "poky eaters." We need slow-flow nipples (many different brands—some try many before settling on the right one), and we need pacing (the mnemonic suck, swallow, breathe), the side-lying position, and a speech therapist to help [20, 21]. Learn how to wean me off supplements in Chap. 6.

The good news is that almost all of us survive (99%) [22]. Our risk for neurodevelopmental delays is higher when compared to term infants [23–27], and the challenges we experience (described above) further impacts our neurodevelopmental outcomes [28–36]. Chapter 9 explains what my brain looks like and how some of the early challenges I face impact my behavior, speech, and ability to learn later in life.

In summary, the heartfelt message we want to leave you with is to please help make our dreams "happen." To my parents and care providers, be responsive to my cues and actions. It will help me realize my full potential. Remember it is a wonderful world somewhere over the rainbow (Israel Kamakawiwo'ole, Hawaiian singer). The world is our oyster. Enjoy us while you can. It is a once-in-a-lifetime experience!!

To my colleagues, this inspiration came to me from somewhere over the rainbow and I want to share with you:

R—recognize and respect our population, the late preterm infant.
A—assess our needs.
I—implement the EBP which is evidence-based practice.
N—nipple us with the slow-flow nipples.
B—bundle our care to allow for rest periods.
O—open communication (consistent and concise information) with my parents will enhance the parent-infant relationship.
W—whole team working together is what it takes to get me home (nurses, midwives, doctors, respiratory therapists, lactation, speech therapist, occupational therapists, physiotherapists, and most important my mom and dad).
S—skin to skin (kangaroo care) is what we love.

Susan Kau BSN RNC-NIC March 22, 2018.

We conclude this book with stories from around the world as globally the care of LPIs varies widely. Our narratives come from Brazil, Japan, Malawi, Russia, and South Africa and tell a very personal story about caring for this unique population—late preterm infants!!

References

1. Kugelman A, Colin AA. Late preterm infants: near term but still in a critical developmental time period. Pediatrics. 2013;132(4):741–51. https://doi.org/10.1542/peds.2013-1131.
2. Premji SS, Currie G, Reilly S, Dosani A, Oliver LM, Lodha AK, Young M. A qualitative study: mothers of later preterm infants relate their experiences of community-based care. PLoS One. 2017;12(3):e0174419. https://doi.org/10.1371/journal.pone.0174419.
3. Engle WA, Tomashek KM, Wallman C. Committee on Fetus and Newborn, American Academy of Pediatrics. "Late preterm" infants: a population at risk. Pediatrics. 2007;120(6):1390–9.
4. Forsythe ES, Allen PJ. Health risks associated with late-preterm infants: implications for newborn primary care. Pediatr Nurs. 2013;39(4):197–201.
5. Kingston D, Heaman M, Fell D, Dzakpasu S, Chalmers B. Factors associated with perceived stress and stressful life events in pregnant women: findings from the Canadian Maternity Experiences Survey. Matern Child Health J. 2012;16(1):158–68.
6. Priest SR, Austin MP, Barnett BB, Buist A. A psychosocial risk assessment model (PRAM) for use with pregnant and postpartum women in primary care settings. Arch Womens Ment Health. 2008;11(5–6):307–17.
7. Rose MS, Pana G, Premji S. Prenatal maternal anxiety as a risk factor for preterm birth and the effects of heterogeneity on this relationship: a systematic review and meta-analysis. Biomed Res Int. 2016;2016:8312158. https://doi.org/10.1155/2016/8312158.
8. Premji SS, Yim IS, Dosani A, Kanji Z, Sulaiman S, Musana JW, Samia P, Shaikh K, Letourneau N, MiGHT Group. Psychobiobehavioral model for preterm birth in pregnant women in low- and middle-income countries. BioMed Res Int. 2015;2015:450309. https://doi.org/10.1155/2015/450309.
9. Hawes K, McGowan E, O'Donnell M, Tucker R, Vohr B. Social emotional factors increase risk of postpartum depression in mothers of preterm infants. J Pediatr. 2016;179:61–7. https://doi.org/10.1016/j.jpeds.2016.07.008.

10. Samra HA, Dutcher J, McGrath JM, Foster M, Klein L, Djira G, Hansen J, Wallenburg D. Effect of skin-to-skin holding on stress in mothers of late-preterm infants: a randomized controlled trial. Adv Neonatal Care. 2015;15(5):354–64. https://doi.org/10.1097/ANC.0000000000000223.

11. Sisson H, Jones C, Williams R, Lachanudis L. Metaethnograhic synthesis of fathers' experience of the neonatal intensive care unit environment during hospitalization of their premature Infant. J Obstet Gynecol Neonat Nurs. 2015;44(4):471–80. https://doi.org/10.1111/1552-6909.12662.

12. Reuter S, Moser C, Baack M. Respiratory distress in the newborn. Pediatr Rev. 2014;35(10):417–29. https://doi.org/10.1542/pir.35-10-417.

13. Hunt CE. Ontogeny of autonomic regulation in late preterm infant born at 34–37 weeks postmenstrual age. Semin Perinatol. 2006;30(2):73–6. https://doi.org/10.1053/j.semperi.2006.02.005.

14. Adamkin DH, Committee on Fetus and Newborn. Clinical report-postnatal glucose homeostasis in late-preterm and term infants. Pediatrics. 2011;127(3):575–9.

15. Crenshaw JT. Healthy birth practice #6: keep mother and baby together – it's best for mother, baby, and breastfeeding. J Perinat Educ. 2014;23(4):211–7. https://doi.org/10.1891/1058-1243.23.4.211.

16. Darcy AE. Complications of the late preterm infant. J Perinat Neonatal Nurs. 2009;23(1):78–86. https://doi.org/10.1097/HPN.0b013e31819685b6.

17. Boyle EM, Field DJ, Wolke D, Alfirevic Z. Effects of gestational age at birth on health outcomes at 3 and 5 years of age: population based cohort study. BMJ. 2012;344:e896. https://doi.org/10.1136/bmj.e89.

18. Dong Y, Yu JL. An overview of morbidity, mortality and long-term outcome of late preterm birth. World J Pediatr. 2011;7(3):199–204. https://doi.org/10.1007/s12519-011-0290-8.

19. Harron K, Gilbert R, Cromwell D, Oddie S, van der Meulen J. Newborn length of stay and risk of readmission. Paediatr Perinat Epidemiol. 2017;31(3):221–32. https://doi.org/10.1111/ppe.12359.

20. Meierr PP, Furman LM, Degenhardt M. Increased lactation risk for late preterm infants and mothers: evidence and management strategies to protect breastfeeding. J Midwifery Womens Health. 2007;52(6):579–87. https://doi.org/10.1016/j.jmwh.2007.08.003.

21. Shaker CS. Cue-based co-regulated feeding in the neonatal intensive care unit: supporting parents in learning to feed their preterm infant. Newborn Infant Nurs Rev. 2013;13(1):1–55.

22. Allen MC, Cristofalo EA, Kim C. Outcomes of preterm infants: morbidity replaces mortality. Clin Perinatol. 2011;38:441–54.

23. Klebanoff MA, Keim SA. Epidemiology: the changing face of preterm birth. Clin Perinatol. 2011;38(3):339–50.

24. Tomashek KM, Shapiro-Mendoza CK, Davidoff MJ, Petrini JR. Differences in mortality between late-preterm and term singleton infants in the United States, 1995–2002. J Pediatr. 2007;151:450–6.

25. Khashu M, Narayanan M, Bhargava S, Osiovich H. Perinatal outcomes associated with preterm birth at 33 to 36 weeks' gestation: a population-based cohort study. Pediatrics. 2009;23:109–13.

26. Shapiro-Mendoza CK, Tomashek KM, Kotelchuck M, Barfield W, Nannini A, Weiss J, Declercq E. Effect of late-preterm birth and maternal medical conditions on newborn morbidity risk. Pediatrics. 2008;121:e223–32.

27. Visruthan NK, Agarwal P, Sriram B, Rajadurai VS. Neonatal outcome of the late preterm infant (34 to 36 weeks): the Singapore story. Ann Acad Med Singap. 2015;44:235–43.

28. Walker M. Breastfeeding management for the late preterm infant: practical interventions for "little imposters". Clin Lact. 2010;1:22–6.

29. Medoff-Cooper B, Bilker W, Kaplan J. Sucking behavior as a function of gestational age: a cross-sectional study. Infant Behav Dev. 2001;24:83–94.

30. Bakewell-Sachs S. Near-term/late preterm infants. Newborn Infant Nurs Rev. 2007;7:68–71.

31. Laptook A, Jackson GL. Cold stress and hypoglycemia in the late preterm ("near-term") infant: impact on nursery of admission. Semin Perinatol. 2006;30:24–7.

32. The American Academy of Breastfeeding Medicine (2011). ABM clinical protocol #10: breastfeeding the late preterm infant ($34^{0/7}$–$36^{6/7}$ weeks gestation) (First Revision June 2011). Breastfeed Med. 2011;6:151–6.
33. Baker B. Evidence-based practice to improve outcomes for late preterm infants. J Obstet Gynecol Neonatal Nurs. 2015;44:127–34.
34. Gouyon JB, Iacobelli S, Ferdynus C, Bonsante F. Neonatal problems of late and moderate preterm infants. Semin Fetal Neonatal Med. 2012;17:146–52.
35. Wang ML, Dorer DJ, Fleming MP, Catlin EA. Clinical outcomes of near-term infants. Pediatrics. 2004;114:372–6.
36. Hillman N. Hyperbilirubinemia in the late preterm infant. Newborn Infant Nurs Rev. 2007;7:91–4.

Mother's Physical Health Before Delivery Matters: What Happens and Why?

2

Jennifer Marandola and Gisela Becker

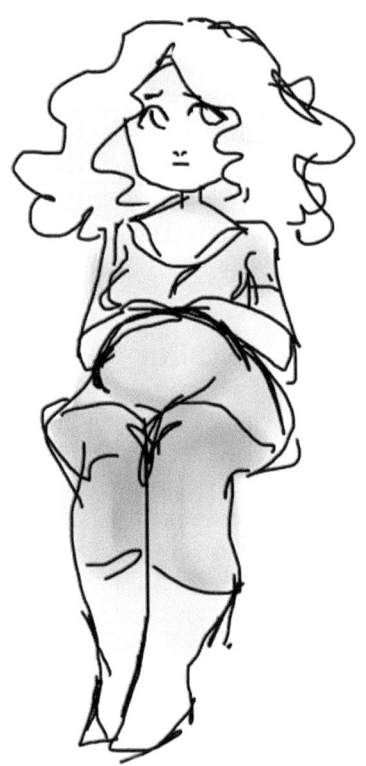

J. Marandola (✉)
volet Jeunesse/Santé-Publique, Centre intégré universitaire de santé et de services sociaux de l'Ouest-de-l'île-de-Montréal, Montréal, QC, Canada

G. Becker
Department of Health and Community Services, Government of Newfoundland and Labrador, St. John's, NL, Canada
e-mail: GiselaBecker@gov.nl.ca

2.1   Introduction

There has been a significant rise in late preterm births globally [1]; it is the leading cause of death in children under the age of 5 years [2]. Disparities in survival rates around the world are glaring. In poor countries, half of the babies born at or below 32 weeks die due to a lack of appropriate care such as warmth, breastfeeding support, and basic care for infections and breathing difficulties. In high-income countries, almost all of these babies survive [3]. The incidence of late preterm delivery and the contribution of multiple pregnancies appear to be growing. Increases in multiple births, obstetric intervention, and improved accuracy of measurement of gestational age have contributed to a rise in the incidence of late preterm delivery [4]. The approach to management of births in the late preterm period varies; it includes health education, health advice, and medical management such as glucocorticoids to decrease the incidence of neonatal respiratory distress syndrome (RDS) [5–8]. Previous findings endorsed imminent delivery if mothers were to go into labor during the late preterm period; however, recent literature has shown that expectant management of labor in the late preterm period is an acceptable alternative to care as compared to immediate delivery [5–7].

2.2   Causes of Late Preterm Birth

The etiology of late preterm births may differ from very preterm deliveries. Contributing factors include indicated interventions due to maternal complications [1, 4]. These complications may include preterm premature rupture of membranes (PPROM), preeclampsia or eclampsia, complicated insulin-dependent diabetes mellitus, or fetal indications such as oligohydramnios and intrauterine growth restriction (IUGR) [1, 4]. IUGR can often result from multiple causes, including infection or inflammation, vascular disease, and uterine overdistension [1, 4].

Late preterm infants have an increased risk to be born by caesarean section because of underlying medical conditions in the mother or infant, such as gestational hypertension, diabetes, placenta previa, and abdominal surgery during pregnancy, but also causes of IUGR and medical concerns in the fetus [9]. More recently, governments and clinicians have expressed concern about the rise in the numbers of caesarean sections and the potential negative consequences for maternal and infant health [10]. Of particular concern is the greater use of elective caesarean section at 36 weeks gestation which contributes to more late preterm births especially when there are no consistent means to exactly confirm the length of the pregnancy [10].

2.3   Induction of Labor

Late preterm births may sometimes result from early induction of labor for medical or nonmedical reasons [3, 11]. The incidence of both gestational and pregestational diabetes is increasing worldwide. Women who develop diabetes in pregnancy usually have healthy pregnancies and babies, but gestational diabetes can cause serious problems, especially if it goes unrecognized, such as increased risk of operative and caesarean deliveries, postpartum hemorrhage, birth trauma, and shoulder dystocia [12]. Maternal hyperglycemia during late gestation is more likely to lead to fetal macrosomia, hypoxia, polycythemia, and cardiomegaly with outflow tract obstruction [13]. Certain medical conditions such as diabetes that develops before the pregnancy must be managed carefully because it is associated with a variety of complications including prematurity and late prematurity [3]. The objective of induction of labor in gestational diabetes and pregestational diabetes pregnancies at 36 to 38 weeks gestation has traditionally been to prevent stillbirth and prevent too much fetal growth and its associated complication [14]. The American College of Obstetricians and Gynecologists (ACOG) does not recommend induced vaginal or planned caesarean delivery prior to 39 weeks gestation unless medically indicated [4]. There is a desire to reduce preterm birth, and with the awareness of the potential complications for late preterm infants, there is also an understanding that some preterm births are necessary for the mother, baby, or both to achieve optimal health outcome [12]. The impact of preterm and late preterm births is more challenging to reduce in low-income countries and cannot be achieved with practice standards of more developed countries. Interventions include adequate access to quality obstetrical and newborn care as well as preventative measures and education [15].

2.4   Immediate Delivery vs Expectant Management

The management of preterm labor includes early diagnosis, identifying the cause of preterm labor and treating the underlying cause when possible, attempting to arrest labor when appropriate, and intervening to reduce neonatal morbidity and mortality [16]. Tocolysis is primarily used to prolong pregnancy for 48 h or more when given before 34 weeks gestation [17]. This is not the case with late preterm labor. Recent literature suggests that expectant management may be more appropriate during the late preterm phase [5–7]. This involves careful monitoring by healthcare professionals including continuous surveillance if rupture of membranes has occurred and occasionally a hospital admission.

Antenatal hospitalization has been linked to increased postpartum depression [18]. As such, a careful consideration of the risks and benefits of hospital admission and monitoring should not only be conducted but discussed with the parents as well. In the late preterm period, feelings of uncertainty and unpreparedness have been shown to plague mothers making them especially vulnerable to advice of healthcare providers [19]. It is essential that healthcare providers discuss the impact of each decision made during the management of labor during this period as well as the effects of those decisions on neonatal outcomes.

Chapter 3: Maternal Emotional Health Before and After Birth Matters examines why emotional health during pregnancy matters. Stress, anxiety, and depression are the most common conditions that women face during pregnancy and the postpartum period. Working with women, their partners, their families, and the wider community supports the reduction of stress, anxiety, and depression in expectant mothers [20].

2.5   The Corticosteroid Debate

Healthcare providers managing women during antenatal hospitalization in the late preterm period or threatened labor during this period must also evaluate the need for administration of corticosteroids [1, 21, 22]. In previous years, antenatal glucocorticoid therapy to accelerate fetal lung maturity was considered until 34 weeks gestation [11, 23]. Corticosteroid treatment use beyond the 34-week mark had been linked to causing unphysiological activation of glucocorticoid receptors in the brain, as well as behavioral changes, and delayed cognitive functioning [24, 25]. Recent practice changes have shown that antenatal glucocorticoid therapy given to women with imminent delivery during the late preterm period can help the newborn by [26] decreasing the need for respiratory support and [2] decreased rate of transient tachypnea, bronchopulmonary dysplasia, and a composite of respiratory distress syndromes [21, 23, 27].

According to new recommendations, a woman who presents in labor within the late preterm period and who has not received a previous dose of corticosteroids should be given a dose if she (1) has a cervix dilation of at least 3 cm or 75% effacement, (2) has preterm premature rupture of membranes, or (3) is at risk of giving birth within the next 7 days [4, 16, 27, 28]. This new recommendation is contradictory to what has previously been a common practice with antenatal corticosteroids and as such has sparked some controversy in different specialties [4, 21, 22]. Literature has begun to emerge assessing the potential impact of extending this recommendation to the late preterm period [4, 21, 22]. An uncertainty continues to exist among healthcare providers as to whether the short-term respiratory benefits of corticosteroids outweigh the long-term adverse outcomes of prolonged and persistent neonatal hypoglycemia [27, 29, 30].

One common side effect of corticosteroids is the induced hyperglycemia in the mother. This induced hyperglycemia begins at about 12 h after the first dose and lasts up to 5 days [1, 16]. For women delivering within this 5-day time frame, and within their hyperglycemic state, their infant may be at greater risk for neonatal hypoglycemia [31], of which the late preterm infant is already at an elevated risk. Why is that? At birth, glucose concentration in newborns is about 80% that of maternal glucose concentration [32]. How does this happen? In utero, fetal glucose concentrations are maintained by diffusion from mother to fetus through the placenta [32]. After the cord is clamped, the newborn learns to produce glucose in the pancreas. In late preterm newborns, this pancreatic glucose regulation is immature, and their glycogen levels are typically lower than term infants and are used up at a faster pace [10, 32]. As such, a mother who might give birth within the 5-day time frame of having received corticosteroids would give birth to a newborn with too much insulin in the blood and potentially exacerbate risk of transitional neonatal hypoglycemia if poorly managed or monitored after birth [31]. The evidence is unclear however whether the new recommendation puts these infants at greater risk of neonatal hypoglycemia and hyperbilirubinemia [31]. Antenatal corticosteroid studies performed on populations ≥37 weeks have not had the same results of increased hypoglycemia or long-term outcomes [33].

Increasingly, late preterm infants are monitored after birth on maternal child units and no longer in intensive care settings. These babies need to demonstrate stable blood glucose levels and adequate feeding and elimination before discharged home [34]. As such, the same studies that recommend the use of antenatal cortico-steroids also recommend that hospitals have in place a hypoglycemia protocol that includes management and monitoring of late preterm infants [16, 22, 29, 30]. Careful counseling and discussion of risks and benefits of this recommendation are needed with parents when considering extending antenatal corticosteroid recom-mendation to the late preterm population.

2.6   Hypoglycemia in the Late Preterm Infant

Given discussion of corticosteroids and management of gestational diabetes in pregnancy, it is important that there be added emphasis on the high risk of transi-tional hypoglycemia that can occur for the late preterm infant. Hypoglycemia is one of the most common transition challenges, occurring in at least 15.6% of late preterm infants and at a rate three times higher than term newborns [35]. Late pre-term infants, like premature infants, are more likely to develop hypoglycemia; they have limited glycogen stores and immature liver function [32]. Extending the use of corticosteroids may increase the risk of hypoglycemia as some of these babies are born to diabetic mothers, are small for gestational age, and/or are growth-restricted [4, 28].

During transition to extra-uterine life, newborn glucose levels fall to its lowest level at about 30–90 min after birth and can stay low for the first 4 h [32]. In late preterm newborns, this nadir is 1.7–2.2 mmol/L [17]. Late preterm infants are par-ticularly at risk for rebound and recurrent hypoglycemia [32]. Rebound hypoglyce-mia is defined as an episode of hypoglycemia within 6 h after successful treatment, and recurrent hypoglycemia is defined as further episodes of hypoglycemia after successful treatment, within 48 h after birth [32, 35].

The newborn brain depends on blood glucose as its main source of fuel. Too little glucose may impair the brain's ability to function; severe or prolonged hypoglyce-mia may result in seizures and serious brain injury [32, 35, 36].

Glucose levels can drop if:
1. There is too much insulin in the blood.
2. The baby is not producing enough glucose.
3. The baby's body is using more glucose than is being produced.
4. The baby is not able to feed enough to keep glucose levels up [32, 35].

Transient hypoglycemia in the first hours after birth is common and is part of adaptation to postnatal life [35, 36]. Transient, single, brief periods of hypoglycemia are unlikely to cause permanent neurological damage [32, 35, 36]. Persistent or prolonged periods of hypoglycemia, particularly when symptoms are present, may lead to neurological impairment of the newborn [32, 35, 36]. However, there currently exists no evidence that can answer:

1. How low a glucose concentration is too low?
2. What glucose concentration causes brain damage?
3. How long can it be low before we encounter irreversible brain damage [30, 32, 35, 36]?

The management of hypoglycemia in late preterm infants includes monitoring the overall metabolic and physiologic status of the baby without unnecessarily disrupting the mother–infant relationship [30, 35]. Communication with the responsible healthcare provider regarding the newborn's evolving health status must be maintained to ensure safe care.

2.7 Conclusion

Maternal management impacts the late preterm birth; thus a skilled midwife or healthcare provider is critical for appropriate provision of care to both the mother (during and after delivery) and late preterm infant. Causes and management of late premature birth continue to vary in recommendations of induction of labor, intermittent delivery versus expectant management, the use of antenatal glucocorticoid therapy to accelerate fetal lung maturity, and management of gestational diabetes in pregnancy. This chapter aimed to clarify factors contributing to the late preterm birth and discusses current maternal and infant standard and trends in a variety of settings. It placed emphasis on the limited amount of research and evidence available for management of both the mother and infant during this time period and that the late preterm population continues to be an area where further recommendations and guidelines are needed. Given the limited evidence available, providers must anticipate challenges in late preterm infants when counseling parents on management of labor and follow current and evidence-informed protocols for successful treatment without unnecessarily disrupting the mother–infant relationship.

References

1. Miracle X, Di Renzo GC, Stark A, Fanaroff A, Carbonell-Estrany X, Saling E. Coordinators of world association of perinatal medicine (WAPM) prematurity group guidelines for the use of antenatal corticosteroids for fetal maturation. J Perinat Med. 2008;36:191–6.
2. Statistics Canada. Preterm live births in Canada, 2000 to 2013. https://www.statcan.gc.ca/pub/82-625-x/2016001/article/14675-eng.htm. Accessed 17 Oct 2017.

3. World Health organization (WHO). Preterm birth. 2017. http://www.who.int/mediacentre/factsheets/fs363/en/. Accessed 2 Feb 2018.
4. Souter V, Kauffman E, Marshall A, Katon J. Assessing the potential impact of extend-ing antenatal steroids to the late preterm period. Am J Obstet Gynecol. 2017;217(461):e1–7.
5. Lim J, Allen V, Scott H, Allen A. Late preterm delivery in women with preterm prelabour rupture of membranes. J Obstet Gynecol Can. 2010;32(6):555–60.
6. Melamed N, Klinger G, Tenenbaum-Gavish K, Herscovici T, Linder N, Hod M, Yogev Y. Short-term neonatal outcome in low-risk, spontaneous, singleton, late preterm deliveries. Obstet Gynecol. 2009;114(2):253–60.
7. Quist-Nelson J, de Ruigh A, Seidler A, van der Ham D, Willekes C, Berghella V, et al. Immediate delivery compared with expectant management in late preterm prelabor rupture of membranes. Obstet Gynecol. 2018;0(0):1–11.
8. American Congress of Obstetricians and Gynecologists (ACOG). Practice bulletin: management of preterm labor. Obstet Gynecol. 2016;128:e155–64.
9. Society of Obstetricians and Gynaecologists of Canada (SOGC). ALARM course manual, chapter 18: preterm labour and preterm birth. 23rd ed. Ottawa, ON: SOGC; 2017.
10. Lockwood CJ. Overview of preterm labor and delivery. UpToDate. Waltham, MA: UpToDate, Inc; 2012.
11. White DE, Fraser-Lee NJ, Tough S, Newburn-Cook CV. The content of prenatal care and its relationship to preterm birth in Alberta, Canada. Health Care Women Int. 2006;27(9):777–92.
12. Spong CY, Mercer BM, D'Alton M, Kilpatrick S, Blackwell S, Saade G. Timing of indicated late-preterm and early-term birth. National Institute of Child Health and Human Development. Obstet Gynecol. 2011;118(2 Pt 1):323–33. https://doi.org/10.1097/AOG.0b013e3182255999.
13. Mitanchez D, Yzydorczyk C, Simeoni U. What neonatal complications should the pediatrician be aware of in case of maternal gestational diabetes? World J Diabetes. 2015;6(5):734–43. https://doi.org/10.4239/wjd.v6.i5.734.. PMCID: PMC4458502
14. SOGC. Policy statement: maternal transport policy. J Obstet Gynaecol Can. 2005;27(10):956–8.
15. Morisaki N, Togoobaatar G, Vogel JP, Souza JP, Rowland Hogue CJ, Jayaratne K, Ota E, Mori R. WHO multicountry survey on maternal and newborn health research network: risk factors for spontaneous and provider-initiated preterm delivery in high and low human development index countries: a secondary analysis of the World Health Organization multi-country survey on maternal and newborn health. BJOG. 2014;121(Suppl 1):101–9. https://doi.org/10.1111/1471-0528.12631.
16. Booker W, Gyamfi-Bannerman C. Antenatal corticosteroids: who should we be treating? Clin Perinatol. 2018;45(2):181–98. https://doi.org/10.1016/j.clp.2018.01.002.
17. Wright N, Marinelli KA, The Academy of Breastfeeding Medicine. ABM protocol #1: guidelines for glucose monitoring and treatment of hypoglycemia in term and late preterm neonates. Breastfeed Med. 2014;9(4):173–9.
18. Byatt N, Hicks-Courant K, Davidson A, Levesque R, Mick E, Allison J, Moore-Simas TA. Depression and anxiety among high-risk obstetric inpatients. Gen Hosp Psychiatry J. 2014;35(2):112–6. https://doi.org/10.1016/j.genhosppsych.2012.11.006.
19. Brandon D, Tully K, Silva S, Malcolm W, Murtha A, Turner B, Holditch-Davis D. Emotional responses of mothers of late preterm and term infants. J Obstet Gynecol Neonatal Nurs. 2011;40:719–31. https://doi.org/10.1111/j.1552-6909.2011.01290.x.
20. Bright K, Becker G. Maternal emotional health before and after birth matters. In: Premji SS, editor. Late preterm infants. A guide for nurses, clinicians and allied health professionals. New York: Springer; 2018.
21. Gyamfi-Bannerman C, et al. Antenatal betamethasone for women at risk for late preterm delivery. N Engl J Med. 2016;374(14):1311–20. https://doi.org/10.1056/NEJMoa1516783.
22. Society for Maternal-Fetal Medicine (SMFM). Implementation of the use of antenatal corticosteroids in the late preterm birth period in women at risk for preterm delivery. Am J Obstet Gynecol. 2016;215(2):B14. https://doi.org/10.1016/j.ajog.2016.03.013.
23. Wapner R, Gyamfi-Bannerman C, Thom E. What we have learned about antenatal corticosteroid regimens. Semin Perinatol. 2016;40:291–7.

24. Smith GC, Rowitch D, Mol BW. The role of prenatal steroids at 34–36 weeks of gestation. Arch Dis Child Fetal Neonatal Ed. 2017;102:F284.
25. Chang YP. Evidence for the adverse effect of perinatal glucocorticoid use on the developing brain. Korean J Pediatr. 2014;57:101.
26. Canadian Premature Babies Foundation. Premature birth in Canada: an environmental scan–final report, 2014. http://cpbf-fbpc.org/wp-content/uploads/2017/05/2014-07-23-CPBF-Premature-Birth-environmental-scan_Final.pdf. Accessed 18 Oct 2017.
27. Nowik C, Davies G, Smith G. We should proceed with caution when it comes to antenatal corticosteroids after 34 weeks. J Obstet Gynecol Can. 2017;39(1):49–51.
28. Kalra S, Kalra B, Gupta Y. Glycemic management after antenatal corticosteroid therapy. North Am J Med Sci. 2014;6(2):71–6. https://doi.org/10.4103/1947-2714.127744.
29. Crowther C, Harding J. Antenatal glucocorticoids for late preterm birth? N Engl J Med. 2016;374(14):1376–7.
30. Adamkin DH. Committee on fetus and newborn. Clinical report-postnatal glucose homeostasis in late-preterm and term infants. Pediatrics. 2011;127(3):575–9.
31. Pettit K, Tran S, Lee E, Caughey A. The association of antenatal corticosteroids with neonatal hypoglycemia and hyperbilirubinemia. J Matern Fetal Neonatal Med. 2014;27(7):1476–4954. https://doi.org/10.3109/14767058.2013.832750.
32. Garg M, Devaskar S. Glucose metabolism in the late preterm infant. Clin Perinatol. 2006;33:853–70.
33. Saccone G, Berghella V. Antenatal corticosteroids for maturity of term or near term fetuses: systematic review and meta-analysis of randomized controlled trials. Br Med J. 2016;355:i5044.
34. Csont GL, Groth S, Hopkins P, Guillet R. An evidence-based approach to breastfeeding neonates at risk for hypoglycemia. J Obstet Gynecol Neonatal Nurs. 2014;3:71–81. https://doi.org/10.1111/1552-6909.12272.
35. Wright J, Fowler Byers J, Norris A. Factors related to birth transition success of late preterm infants. Elsevier Newborn Infant Nurs Rev. 2012;12(2):97–105. https://doi.org/10.1053/j.nainr.2012.03.009.
36. Adamkin PH. Postnatal glucose homeostasis in late preterm and term infants. Committee on fetus and newborn. Pediatrics. 2011;127:575–9.

Maternal Emotional Health Before and After Birth Matters

3

Katherine Bright and Gisela Becker

3.1 Introduction

Stress, anxiety, and depression are the most common mental health problems that women face during pregnancy and the postpartum period [1]. One in four women experience anxiety or depression during their pregnancy making emotional health issues one of the top three pregnancy complications [2, 3]. While women are routinely assessed for other less common problems, most healthcare professionals do not screen or assess women for emotional health problems during pregnancy and postpartum period [3]. Women's emotional health during pregnancy and after birth matters. The impact of maternal stress, anxiety, and depression during pregnancy and the postpartum period has significant short- and long-term consequences for women, children, and families.

Mothers of infants born prematurely are reported to have depression rates of 28–40% during their stay in the neonatal intensive care unit (NICU) and the early postpartum period [4]. Their vulnerability to postpartum depression is associated with previous mental health concerns, the stress around the preterm birth, concerns about their infant's health, the NICU experience, and disrupted attainment of the maternal role [5]. The experiences of mothers of late preterm infants are complicated by early delivery and maternal and infant health concerns resulting in

Special thanks to Dr. Sheri-Lynn Cassity, M.D., F.R.C.P.C., for her comprehensive review and thoughtful feedback on this chapter.

K. Bright (✉)
Faculty of Nursing, University of Calgary, Calgary, AB, Canada

Women's Mental Health Clinic, Alberta Health Services, Calgary, AB, Canada
e-mail: ksbright@ucalgary.ca; Katherine.Bright@albertahealthservices.ca

G. Becker
Department of Health and Community Services, Government of Newfoundland and Labrador, St. John's, NF, Canada
e-mail: GiselaBecker@gov.nl.ca

significant emotional distress in these women. The emotional distress of mothers of late preterm infants changes over time and impacts parenting, infant health, and child development [6].

3.2 Why Maternal Emotional Health During Pregnancy Matters

3.2.1 Maternal Emotional Health: Impact on Pregnancy

Stress, anxiety, and depression during pregnancy can disrupt the underlying physiological stress response in women [7]. While stressors may vary from major life events to hassles of daily life, the whole stress regulatory system is activated [8]. The stress regulatory system consists of the hypothalamus–pituitary–adrenal cortex system (HPA axis) and the sympathoadrenal system [8]. Following activation of the stress response system, there is a release of various hormones including corticotropin–releasing hormone (CRH), adrenocorticotropin–releasing hormone (ACTH), cortisol, and/or adrenaline into the blood stream [7, 8]. For pregnant women, the stress response to major life events and/or daily obstacles may be compounded by challenges associated with pregnancy-related physical changes, hormonal modifications, and pregnancy-specific anxiety [9]. The HPA axis and pregnancy-related physical changes have a strong impact on women's sexual and reproductive capacities [8, 10]. As a result, stress, anxiety, and depression can have major adverse effects on the in utero environment and consequently on the developing unborn baby [7]. As such, there is increased risk of spontaneous abortion, structural craniofacial malformations, heart defects, preeclampsia in the later phase of pregnancy, preterm delivery including late preterm birth, reduced birth weight, and smaller head size [7, 8, 10].

These high levels of stress, anxiety, and depression during pregnancy are associated with reduced gestation and preterm delivery [11]. When the increase in cortisol occurs at the end of a normal pregnancy, it leads to an increase in uterine activity and ultimately delivery [12]. Unfortunately, when this cascade of events happens too early in the pregnancy, the result is preterm delivery and preeclampsia. Worldwide, preterm births remain a pronounced maternal-child health matter [11, 13–15]. Preterm births are further subdivided into early preterm births (<34 weeks) and later preterm births (34–$36^{6/7}$ weeks [16]). Late preterm births are the largest and fastest growing subcategory of preterm deliveries [17]. Late preterm infants commonly require weeks to months of care in neonatal intensive care units (NICUs) or special care nurseries (SCNs) [18]. The early days after delivery are a crucial time for development of the mother-infant bond [19]. In addition to being separated from their infant, the NICU or SCN stay is often a time of uncertainty and stress for women regarding the prognosis for their infants [19, 20]. While survival rates for preterm infants have improved over the last two decades, neurobehavioral impairments in preterm children have remained unchanged [20].

3.2.2   Maternal Emotional Health: Impact on Fetal Development

Stress hormones impact the developing fetus through three possible mechanisms: (1) a reduction in blood flow to the uterus and fetus; (2) the transplacental transfer of maternal hormones; and (3) the release of placental CHR into the intrauterine environment [8]. The reduction in blood flow to the uterus and fetus is likely due to the impact of corticosteroids and catecholamines on the tone of peripheral blood vessels [8]. The reduction in blood flow to the uterus and fetus may play a significant role in fetal growth restriction [7, 8, 21]. Maternal hormones, specifically cortisol, cross the placenta such that a small increase in maternal cortisol results in a significant increase in fetal cortisol [8]. The secretion of placental CRH to the intrauterine environment results in an increase in fetal cortisol which affects maturation of all fetal organs [8, 12]. The overproduction of fetal cortisol may restrict development of the fetal nervous system. Damage to the programming/organization of the fetal neuroendocrine system results in impaired neurodevelopment and cognitive and behavioral problems [8, 22–24].

3.2.3   Maternal Emotional Health: Impact on Child Development

As a result of separation after delivery, late preterm infants are reported to be less attentive and responsive in their communication with their mothers [25]. Additionally, preterm birth impairs the mother's opinion of her ability to "mother" her newborn [26]. Understandably, these early days are filled with uncertainty that further adds to maternal emotional distress resulting in increased symptoms of depression and post-traumatic stress disorder (PTSD) [27, 28]. In mothers of term infants, depression and PTSD in the postpartum period significantly impacts maternal sensitivity and maternal-infant attachment [29]. The outcome of sensitive and responsive parenting is shown to increase cognitive, social, and emotional measures for term infants [30]. Insensitive and unresponsive parenting are related to poor regulatory control in infancy and increased psychological problems in adolescence and adulthood [31]. Sensitive and responsive mothering is likely even more important for late preterm infants in order for these children to achieve comparable cognitive, social, and emotional outcomes with term infants [32].

Late preterm infants are a unique group of infants with a number of physical challenges during the early postpartum period [33]. The immature brain of the late preterm infants affects their ability to coordinate behavioral responses to interact with the mother. Because of their immature and unstable behavioral organization, late preterm infants are likely to have a more difficult temperament and lower thresholds for stimulation [34]. Additionally, mothers of late preterm infants are more inclined to experience emotional distress, disrupted sleep patterns, and lower levels of self-confidence [35]. The combination of the immature brains of late preterm infants and maternal difficulties further contributes to their difficulties responding interacting, bonding, and attaching [34].

Maternal sensitivity is attributed to maternal-infant attachment [36]. Attachment theory is considered one of the most useful and important frameworks for understanding how individuals cope with and adjust to life's problems [37]. Bowlby [38] concluded that attachment motives influence how individuals think, feel, and behave in relationships. Attachment styles are largely formed from early childhood experiences with one's primary caregiver [39]. In childhood, these working models represent the individual's attempts to gain solace and security [40]. Individuals compile a mental record of their success at obtaining adequate comfort and support from their parents and later from their relationships with friends and romantic partners [41]. These mental records are abstracted into general beliefs and expectations, essentially working models of the world, significant others, and oneself. These working models are influenced by others' emotional availability and responsiveness to the individual's needs [39, 40]. Mothers of secure infants have interactions with their infants that are more reliable, consistent, sensitive, and accepting of their infants [18, 36].

There is compelling evidence that poor maternal prenatal emotional health can predispose the child to behavioral problems [42]. Increased prenatal stress influences fetal brain growth as suggested by reduced head circumference and lower infant scores on neonatal neurological examination [43]. Preterm births are associated with disruption in brain development that persists into later childhood and adolescence [19]. Additionally, prenatal stress, anxiety, and depression predict various conditions (heart and vascular diseases, adult-onset diabetes, metabolic syndrome) and permanent changes to the HPA axis in the infant [22]. These physiological changes may render the infant/child vulnerable to emotional and cognitive developmental problems, including internalizing and externalizing behaviors (IEBs) [22]. Boys and girls exposed to the same prenatal adversities are prone to different IEBs: girls exhibit more internalizing behaviors (anxiety, depression, sadness), while boys exhibit more externalizing behaviors (aggression, hyperactivity) [44]. Preterm children are more prone to neurodevelopmental, cognitive, and behavioral problems during their infancy and childhood than term counterparts [45]. After delivery, poor maternal emotional mental health can negatively affect bonding with the infant and may result in an increased risk of insecure attachment with ensuing cognitive, attentional, and emotional problems [46–48].

3.2.4   Maternal Emotional Health: Impact on the Postpartum Period

Two decades of research has produced robust evidence that untreated emotional and mental health problems during pregnancy and the postpartum period are associated with negative consequences for women and their families. For many women, depression, anxiety, and stress during pregnancy may continue [49]. Approximately 95% of women who experience depression, anxiety, and stress during their postpartum period reported that their symptoms started in pregnancy [49]. Of those, 41% of women will continue to experience high emotional distress at one year postpartum [50]. Without treatment, 40% of these women with postpartum depression and/or anxiety will continue to have symptoms when their child begins kindergarten [51–53]. After childbirth, prenatal anxiety has been associated with general emotional instability, perceptions of negative birth experiences, and a feeling of personal failure [54, 55].

Mothers of late preterm infants are particularly vulnerable to psychological distress during the perinatal periods [56]. These mothers are reported to be at increased risk of stress and depression, poor sleep, and a decreased sense of competence and well-being during the postpartum period [34]. These maternal challenges coupled with the late preterm infants' tendency toward more difficult temperaments and lower thresholds for stimulation may lead to alterations in attachment, growth, and development [57].

3.2.5   Maternal Emotional Health: Impact on Family Relationships

Becoming a parent or expanding the family with another baby is an important life event for women and their partners [58]. As such, the stress, anxiety, and depression that negatively impacts a woman's ability to function also impacts her personally and her relationship with her partner [59]. In addition to pressure on the relationship and poor partner satisfaction, there is the potential for a lack of intimacy and sexual problems [60]. Poor relationships may result in withdrawal of social support. Severe and prolonged relationship issues may result in separation or divorce [61]. Partner relationship quality is strongly associated with women's emotional distress in pregnancy [58]. Moreover, there is a correlation between paternal depression and maternal depression, with paternal depression occurring more frequently in cases where maternal depression is severe [62] or when they are parenting a medically fragile infant [63].

In addition to depression, fathers of late preterm infants struggle with more stress and anxiety than fathers of term infants [56]. Although emotional health struggles are different for mothers and fathers of late preterm infants, they both contribute to limiting the quality and quantity of serve and return interactions with their infants [56]. These reciprocal interactions between parents and their infants are essential in developing healthy brain architecture development and behavioral development [64]. Late preterm infant's characteristics combined with high parenting stress are barriers to establishing rich and early learning experiences that promote healthy brain development and lay the foundation for optimal neurological, behavioral, and cognitive development [56, 64].

3.3   Maternal Emotional Health Difficulties Commonly Experienced During Pregnancy

3.3.1   Stress During Pregnancy

Stress is defined as any emotional or physical demand on the mind or body—including pregnancy, childbirth, participation in a running race, or battling a disease—which produces either an actual or anticipated disruption of an individual's homeostasis and internal balance [65]. Homeostasis is the body's way of

Table 3.1 Perinatal stress signs and symptoms adapted with permission from https://reproductivementalhealth.ca/ and [42]

Perinatal stress signs and symptoms
Hard to wind/calm down
Difficult to relax
State of nervous energy
Upset easily by trivial things
Agitated
Irritable
Difficulties tolerating interruptions

maintaining a relatively stable condition while adapting to various internal and external environmental factors [65].

When a physical or cognitive stressor is perceived or anticipated, a physiological stress response is initiated to manage the stressor and restore homeostasis. Common signs and symptoms of stress during the perinatal period are found in Table 3.1 (adapted with permission from https://reproductivementalhealth.ca/ and [42]).

3.3.2   Anxiety During Pregnancy

Prenatal anxiety and fear are the presence of those states during pregnancy [66]. Though prenatal anxiety has unique factors, such as extreme hormonal fluctuations, that set it apart from other anxiety states, it is not recognized independently as an anxiety disorder. The Diagnostic and Statistical Manual of Mental Disorders—Fifth Edition (DSM-5; American Psychiatric Association, [67]) acknowledges prenatal anxiety under the "umbrella" of perinatal anxiety. This designation is in relation to anxiety's comorbidity with a major depressive episode in the postpartum period (e.g., peripartum onset) or with an adjustment disorder (e.g., becoming a parent) [68].

In pregnancy, there is an increased rate of anxiety disorders—in particular, generalized anxiety disorder [69]. Also, there is a considerable distinction between the anxiety experienced during pregnancy and that which is not explained by symptoms of general anxiety or comorbid depression [70]. Like other types of anxious and fearful states, prenatal anxiety and fear can be triggered by a diversity of stimuli including labor pain, surgical procedures, and lack of control over body or environment [68, 71, 72].

While pregnancy is a normal health condition, it manifests in physical and physiological changes including weight gain, dizziness, and hormonal fluctuations that are abnormal outside of pregnancy [73]. These changes can act as antecedents, triggering anxiety responses. Studies show that levels of prenatal anxiety fluctuate throughout pregnancy, which indicates that the presence of anxiety should be assessed multiple times across that period [74, 75]. There are several measures to assess prenatal anxiety; many are described and evaluated in Wenzel and Stuart [46]. Many assessments can give false-positive scores due to overlap in somatic symptoms associated with both pregnancy and anxiety. Common signs and symptoms of anxiety during the perinatal period are included in Table 3.2 (adapted with permission from https://reproductivementalhealth.ca/ and [42]). As previously mentioned, some pregnancy symptoms such as hyperventilation, fatigue, insomnia, chest tightness, and gastrointestinal problems also are symptomatic of anxiety. Furthermore, this commonality can lead to false interpretations of anxiety and fear pathology by caregivers and the women themselves [46, 76, 77].

3.3.3   Depression During Pregnancy

Depression is a common disorder that affects one in five women during their lifetime with the greatest prevalence being during the perinatal period [78]. Depression during pregnancy is one of the most common psychiatric disorders in pregnancy and is a serious health problem for women, their partners, and the developing fetus [79]. Common signs and symptoms of depression during the perinatal period are included in Table 3.3 (adapted with permission from https://reproductivemental-health.ca/ and [42]).

Table 3.2 Perinatal anxiety signs and symptoms adapted with permission from https://reproductivementalhealth.ca/ and [42]

Perinatal anxiety signs and symptoms
Feeling fearful, upset, or on guard
Feeling on edge
Feeling irritable
Overdoing activities like washing or cleaning
Difficulties concentrating or poor memory
Feeling restlessness
Having shortness of breath
Having racing/pounding heart
Feeling dizziness, light-headedness, or headaches
Unrealistic ideas or excessive worry about the pregnancy, delivery, or baby

Table 3.3 Perinatal depression signs and symptoms adapted with permission from https://reproductivementalhealth.ca/ and [42]

Perinatal depression signs and symptoms
Feeling depressed or very sad
Feeling hopeless or overwhelmed
Feeling sad most of the day or crying for no reason
Feeling irritable or angry
Feeling guilty or worthless
Feeling restless or low energy
Sleeping more or less than usual
Eating more or less than usual
Withdrawing or isolating from friends or family
Difficulties making decisions or concentrating
Crying for no outward reason
Thoughts of being a 'bad' or 'terrible' mother
Thoughts of harm to self or the baby

The risk for depression in pregnancy is highest among first-time mothers [78]. This relationship is attributed to maternal insecurities, inexperience, fear of childbirth, and adaptation considerations regarding the impact a child has on one's maternal and spousal relationship and change [78]. For women who had experienced emotional and mental health concerns prior to pregnancy, 35.7% experienced depression during their pregnancy [80].

3.4 Identification and Management of Maternal Emotional Health

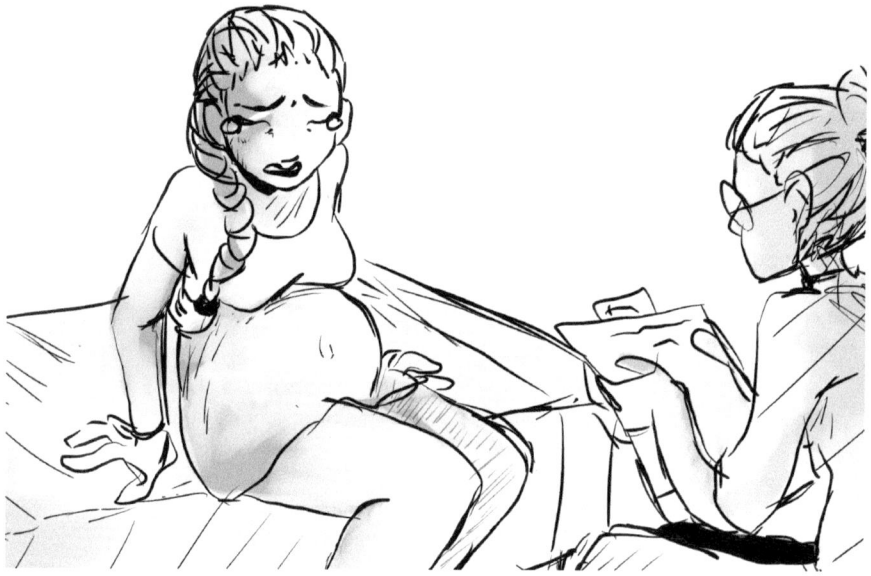

For many healthcare professionals, assessing emotional health during the perinatal period is intimidating. There are many questions such as what to ask, when to ask, and what do you do when someone discloses emotional health concerns. Ultimately, providers want to give best-practice advice for women with emotional/mental health problems during their pregnancy and postpartum period. Given the impact that maternal emotional and mental health has on women, pregnancy, the developing fetus, infants, children, and partners, there is a need and responsibility for timely and appropriate assessment, referral, and intervention.

Women who have emotional health concerns may be reluctant to disclose or discuss their concerns with their healthcare providers. One may fear stigma, being perceived as a "bad mother," or worry that the baby may be taken away. Women may also feel that there is no time or space for them provided to reveal their conditions. They may not feel comfortable sharing their emotional health concerns the first time they are asked, making it important to ask women about their emotional health at each visit. Continuity of care and seeing the same provider(s) may also increase women's ability to speak about their emotional health concerns.

The World Health Organization (WHO) (2015) launched Thinking Healthy, an instructional manual to guide psychosocial management of perinatal mental health concerns [81]. The Thinking Healthy manual articulates that while maternal well-being is universally understood, there are unique differences between high-income countries and developing countries. Approximately 20% of mothers in developing countries experience postpartum mental health concerns; this is close to double the percentage of women in developing countries [81]. In addition to these international guidelines, the United Kingdom National Institute for Health and Care Excellence (NICE) has developed pregnancy and postpartum mental health clinical guidelines to assist healthcare professionals in providing high-quality evidence-based care for women with emotional health problems during their pregnancy and postpartum period. The 2017 updated NICE pregnancy/postpartum mental health guidelines include the stepped/tiered care model to provide direction for the focus and treatment of care (Table 3.4 [82]).

3.4.1   Education and Prevention

Healthcare professionals can work to prevent maternal emotional health problems by promoting self-care strategies. The British Columbia Reproductive Mental Health (BC-RMH) has produced a diagram titled NESTS depicting five important

Table 3.4 Stepped/tiered care (adapted from the NICE pregnancy and postpartum mental health clinical guidelines [82])

	Who is responsible for care?	What is the focus?	What do they do?
Step 1	Family physicians, nurses, obstetricians, and midwives	Identification	Assessment
Step 2	Primary care team, behavioural consultant, primary care mental health professionals, therapists	Mild depression and anxiety disorders	Low-intensity support and/or psychological interventions
Step 3	Primary care team, primary care mental health professionals, clinical psychologists/therapists	Moderate to severe depression and anxiety disorder	Medication and/or high-intensity psychological interventions
Step 4	Pregnancy/postpartum mental health specialists—psychology, psychiatry, nursing	Severe mental illness—psychosis, bipolar disorder, schizophrenia, and severe depression	Complex assessment, medication, psychological interventions, combined interventions
Step 5	Psychiatric crisis/emergency assessment team, inpatient care	Risk of life, severe self-neglect	Medication, combined interventions, ECT

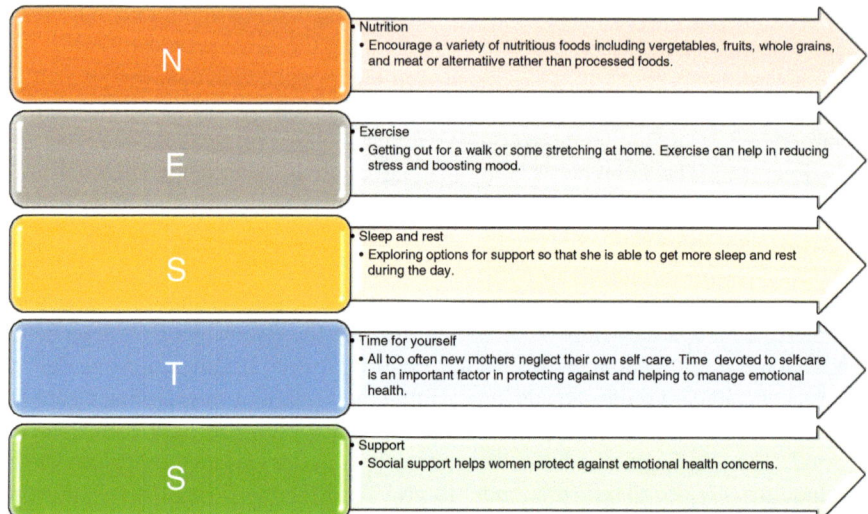

Fig. 3.1 Suggestions for self-care—NESTS—adapted with permission from https://reproductive-mentalhealth.ca/

areas for promoting self-care: nutrition, exercise, sleep/rest, time for yourself, and social support (2014) (Fig. 3.1, adapted from https://reproductivementalhealth.ca/)).

3.4.2 Screening

Assessing frequently, with the same tools allows, healthcare providers the opportunity to note changes over time in stress, anxiety, and depression. This does not mean that women are screened with comprehensive and valid screening tools for stress, anxiety, and depression. Rather, it is prudent to ask women a few probing questions at each visit with their healthcare providers. These questions may be part of a general discussion about women's emotional health during pregnancy and the postpartum period.

3.4.2.1 Quick Screen for Anxiety

Quickly identifying anxiety using the two-item Generalized Anxiety Disorder Scale (GAD-2):

- Over the last 2 weeks, how often have you been bothered by feeling nervous, anxious, or on edge?
  - Not at all (score 0), Several Days (score 1), More than ½ the days (score 2), Nearly every day (score 3).
- Over the last 2 weeks, how often have you been bothered by not being able to stop or control worrying?
  - Not at all (score 0), Several Days (score 1), More than ½ the days (score 2), Nearly every day (score 3).

Scores greater than 3 on the GAD-2 require further investigation using a reliable and valid tool for anxiety screening.

3.4.2.2 Comprehensive Screening for Anxiety

The Perinatal Anxiety Screening Scale (PASS) [83] is a perinatal anxiety screening tool specifically developed to identify a broad range of anxiety symptoms, without the inclusion of overlapping physiological symptoms commonly associated with pregnancy. The PASS was developed to overcome the inadequacies of current assessment tools used to screen for anxiety during pregnancy and the postpartum period [84]. The intent of the PASS is to screen for a broad range of anxiety disorders including problematic symptoms of anxiety during pregnancy and the postpartum period [83]. The PASS is a four-factor compositional screening tool assessing symptoms of (1) acute anxiety and adjustment; (2) general worries and specific fears; (3) perfectionism, control, and trauma; and (4) and social anxiety [83]. Detection of problematic perinatal anxiety is challenging due to variation in the clinical presentation [85]. Although clinicians and researchers agree that screening for perinatal anxiety is necessary, there is little agreement about the most appropriate psychometric tool to use. The PASS was developed to screen for challenging perinatal anxiety and is appropriate for use in antenatal clinics, inpatient/outpatient hospitals, and mental health clinics [83]. The suitability, validity, and usefulness of the PASS make it an essential tool in identifying perinatal anxiety in women [83].

Many general anxiety measures have been used to assess for anxiety in pregnancy without accounting for the physical symptoms of pregnancy. For example, general anxiety tools such as the Hospital Anxiety and Depression Scale (HADS; Zigmond and Snaith [86]), the State-Trait Anxiety Inventory (STAI; Spielberger et al. [87]), and the Beck Anxiety Inventory [88] include physical symptoms that occur in anxiety and pregnancy. The overlap between symptoms of anxiety and pregnancy included in these scales leads to (falsely) elevated anxiety scores [83]. Additionally, instruments such as the Pregnancy Anxiety Scale (PAS; Levin [89]), Pregnancy-Related Anxiety Scale (PRAS; Wadhwa et al. [90]), and Pregnancy-Related Anxiety Questionnaire (PRAQ; Van der Bergh [91]) were developed to measure fears related to labor, pregnancy, and the health/safety of the baby. The PAS, PRAS, and PRAQ have narrow domains with limited range for screening for problematic symptoms of anxiety during pregnancy. These screening tools do not measure the broad range of problematic anxiety symptoms that may occur during the perinatal period. These measures do not indicate the risk of anxiety or specific anxiety disorder symptoms approaching clinical levels [83]. However, the use of assessment tools in clinical practice in high-income and developing countries requires careful consideration of the cultural context, time constrictions, and available resources. For example, the PRAS has face and content validity in studies in developing countries, particularly Tanzania [92]. While these tools may not be able to detect elevated levels of specific anxiety disorders in women during the perinatal period [84], they are effective in assessing a pregnant woman's feelings about her own health, that of her developing fetus, and birth [93].

3.4.2.3 Quickly Screening for Depression

Quickly identifying depression using the Whooley Questions:

- During the past month, how often have you been feeling down, depressed, or hopeless?
- During the past month, have you been often bothered by having little interest or pleasure in doing things?

If women respond positively to either of the depressions identification questions, it is wise to follow up with the Edinburgh Postnatal Depression Scale.

3.4.2.4 Comprehensive Screening for Depression

The Edinburgh Postnatal Depression Scale (EPDS) is a ten-item, self-report questionnaire developed to assist professionals with the identification of depression during the postnatal period [94]. The EPDS was developed to assess postpartum problem experiences that are typically the indicators of depression, such as disturbances in sleep and appetite. This screening tool is routinely administered to women around 6–8 weeks postpartum by their community health nurse or physician. The most consistently reported and recommended postpartum cutoff scores for the EPDS are 9–10 and 12–13 for detecting "possible depression" and "probable depression," respectively [94]. In pregnancy, a higher cutoff of 14–15 is suggested [95]. The EPDS is not as well validated in screening for depression during pregnancy compared to the postpartum period, and the cutoff values differ from the postpartum scores. The original UK study validating the EPDS in pregnancy found that at the 12–13 cutoff score, the EPDS had a sensitivity of 100% for major depression and a specificity of 87%. However, specificity was improved to 96% at the cutoff of 14–15, suggesting a higher cutoff is required to use the EPDS to detect depression in pregnancy [95]. For scores above the clinical cutoff, it is recommended that women be referred to their physician and, if severe emotional health problems are suspected, to a mental health professional [82].

These screening scales *do not confirm a diagnosis* but rather provide a glimpse of the symptoms in that moment and a direction for potential interventions. High screening scores should be reassessed two weeks later. The mental health diagnosis will be determined by the psychiatrist/mental health professional following a full psychiatric assessment [96].

3.5 Interventions

When screening is complete and suggestions for intervention are determined (Table 3.5 ([82–85, 94, 95]), there should be discussion around treatment and prevention options that address concerns for women, their pregnancy, and the fetus or baby. Women need to be made aware of the potential benefits of psychological interventions, psychiatric assessments, and psychotropic medications. During the perinatal period, it should not be assumed that it is always better to go directly to starting psychotropic drugs in perinatal women who are experiencing emotional distress. Women who are already taking psychotropic medications while pregnant or breastfeeding would benefit from

Table 3.5 Screening scales, cut-off points and suggestions for referrals [82–85, 94, 95]

Suggestions for intervention	EPDS scores	The PASS scores
Support (mild anxiety/depression)	8 or less in pregnancy 7 or less in the postpartum period	20 or less
Psychological intervention (mild to moderate anxiety/depression)	9 and above in pregnancy 8 or 11 in the postpartum period	21–40
Psychiatric assessment and intervention (moderate to severe anxiety/depression and/or taking psychotropic medications and considering changing or stopping)	14 and above in pregnancy 12 and above in the postpartum period	41 and above
Emergency psychiatric services	Actively suicidal or at risk for harming baby	Actively suicidal or at risk for harming baby

Any answer other than never on the tenth question of the EPDs requires further investigation of plan, intent to act on plan, and impulsivity to act on plan or new or persistent expression of incompetency as a mother or estrangement from the infant

information and advice about what may occur if treatment is abruptly changed or stopped. Discussions around the use of psychotropic medications need to include: (1) the woman's level of distress from her symptoms being untreated; (2) previous mental health episodes (i.e., severity, responses to treatment, and preference); (3) potential effects of untreated mental health disorders on the fetus or infant; (4) the need for prompt treatment; (5) the risk of fetal abnormalities for pregnant women without a mental disorder; (6) and the possibility of that stopping a medication with known risk during pregnancy might not remove the associated risk [97]. Whenever possible, non-pharmacological treatments should be the primary approach to managing emotional health concerns, but in more severe cases, effective doses of psychotropic medication will be needed after a careful collaborative analysis of the ratio of risk versus benefit.

3.5.1   Support

Support may include peer-mediated support, support groups, and supportive interactions from partners and family members [98]. These social supports play an important role in how individuals manage stress and work through the coping process [99, 100]. Social supports vary in type and can include emotional support, practical help, social companionship, and motivational support [101]. Emotional support is reassurance about self-worth, unconditional positive regard, and the opportunity for confiding [101, 102]. Practical help, also known as instrumental or tangible support, provides direct assistance [101, 103]. Champion [101] also describes the importance of social companionship as a means of engaging in leisure activities. Women struggling with emotional health problems during their pregnancy or postpartum period have indicated that they require practical help from their partners, and emotional and social support from women who have had similar pregnancy and postpartum experiences

[98]. Local prenatal and postpartum peer support groups have been helpful with increasing coping abilities for women with mild symptoms of stress, anxiety, and depression.

3.5.2   Psychological Interventions

Psychological interventions may include but are not limited to cognitive behavioral therapy (CBT), interpersonal psychotherapy (IPT), couples or co-parenting intervention, infant sleep intervention, mindfulness-based cognitive therapy, post-traumatic birth counseling, psychoeducation, and maternal-infant relationship intervention. Such interventions for pregnant and postpartum women should be delivered by competent and capable practitioners [82]. NICE [82] puts forward the recommendation that women with known or suspected emotional health concerns in pregnancy and the postpartum period should be assessed for treatment within two weeks of referral, and psychological interventions should be delivered within one month of the assessment.

3.5.3   Psychiatric Assessment and Intervention

Psychiatric assessments are required when women are struggling with moderate to severe emotional health concerns. The psychiatric assessment will provide clarification around women's diagnosis and treatment options. The greatest benefit for women comes from combining psychological interventions with the psychiatric assessment and intervention [82]. When prescribing psychotropic medication in pregnancy and the postpartum period, the advice from a psychiatric specialist in perinatal emotional health will consider (1) medications with the lowest risk profile for the patient (the mother, the developing fetus, and the baby); (2) the patient's previous response to medication; (3) the lowest effective dose; (4) single medication preference; and (5) the dosage may need to be adjusted during the pregnancy and/or delivery [82].

For healthcare professional and pregnant women, psychotropic medication use in pregnancy must be approached with careful consideration of maternal symptoms of distress and the risk of congenital anomalies associated with fetal exposure to these medications [104]. While there are no psychotropic medications that are completely safe to take during the perinatal period, it is important that women receive enough information to make an informed decision regarding their treatment plan [104]. Information regarding the possible risks and consequences of no treatment as well as the possible risk and harms associated with treatment should be shared with women, their partners, and their families.

3.5.4   Emergency Psychiatric Services

Emergency psychiatric services are required when women are actively suicidal or having active thoughts to harm the fetus or baby. These services are provided through your local emergency department.

Conclusion

Working with women and their partners to reduce stress, anxiety, and depression in expectant mothers can help promote a healthier pregnancy and in utero environment. Given the essential role that maternal emotional health during preg-

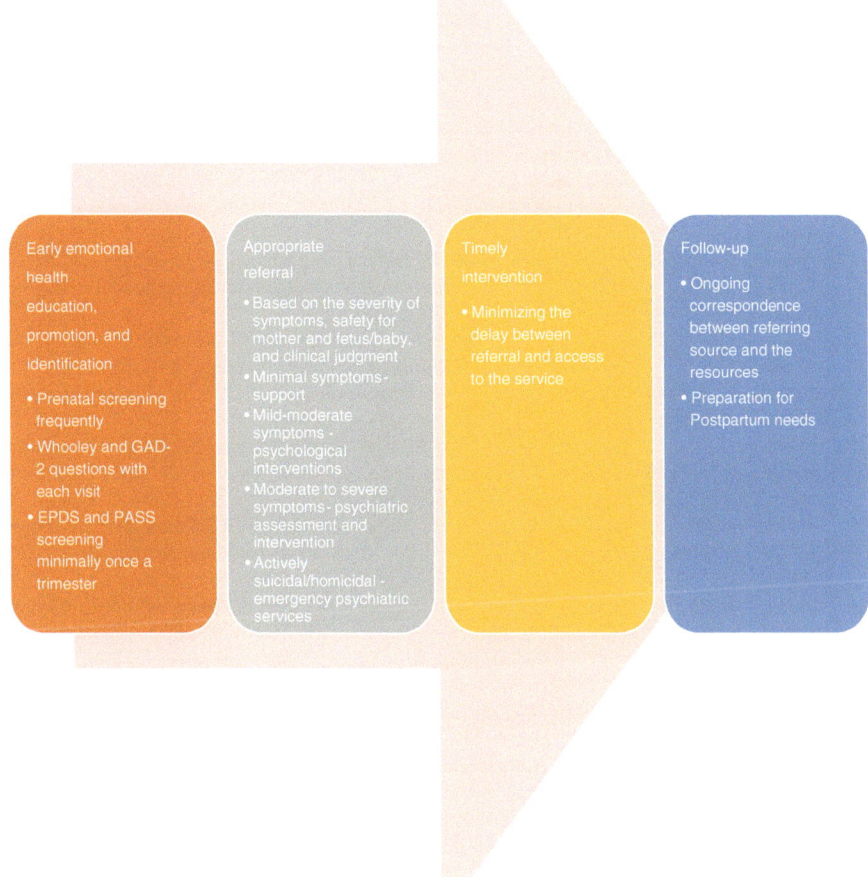

Fig. 3.2 Ideal for perinatal emotional healthcare [82]

nancy play in the long-term health of the developing unborn baby, it is important to identify emotional health concerns early. Stress, anxiety, and depression during the postpartum period are also common and can adversely affect mothers, infants, and families. Regardless of when stress, anxiety, and depression occur during the perinatal period, referral to the most appropriate resources and timely interventions aimed at reducing emotional distress are essential (Fig. 3.2 [82]).

References

1. Milgrom J, Gemmill AW, Bilszta JL, Hayes B, Barnett B, Brooks J, et al. Antenatal risk factors for postnatal depression: a large prospective study. J Affect Disord. 2008;108(1–2):147–57.
2. Kingston D, Heaman M, Fell D, Dzakpasu S, Chalmers B. Factors associated with perceived stress and stressful life events in pregnant women: findings from the Canadian Maternity Experiences Survey. Matern Child Health J. 2012;16(1):158–68.
3. Priest SR, Austin MP, Barnett BB, Buist A. A psychosocial risk assessment model (PRAM) for use with pregnant and postpartum women in primary care settings. Arch Womens Mental Health. 2008;11(5–6):307–17.
4. Hawes K, McGowan E, O'donnell M, Tucker R, Vohr B. Social emotional factors increase risk of postpartum depression in mothers of preterm infants. J Pediatr. 2016;179:61–7.
5. Tahirkheli NN, Cherry AS, Tackett AP, McCaffree MA, Gillaspy SR. Postpartum depression on the neonatal intensive care unit: current perspectives. Int J Womens Health. 2014;6:975.
6. Samra HA, Dutcher J, McGrath JM, Foster M, Klein L, Djira G, et al. Effect of skin-to-skin holding on stress in mothers of late-preterm infants: a randomized controlled trial. Adv Neonatal Care. 2015;15(5):354–64.
7. Isgut M, Smith AK, Reimann ES, Kucuk O, Ryan J. The impact of psychological distress during pregnancy on the developing fetus: biological mechanisms and the potential benefits of mindfulness interventions. J Perinat Med. 2017;31:31.
8. Mulder E, de Medinaa PR, Huizink A, Van den Bergh B, Buitelaar J, Visser G. Prenatal maternal stress: effects on pregnancy and the (unborn) child. Early Hum Dev. 2002;70:3–14.
9. Huizink AC. Prenatal stress and its effect on infant development. Utrecht: Utrecht University Repository; 2001.
10. Andersson L, Sundström-Poromaa I, Wulff M, Åström M, Bixo M. Neonatal outcome following maternal antenatal depression and anxiety: a population-based study. Am J Epidemiol. 2004;159(9):872–81.
11. McDonald SW, Kingston D, Bayrampour H, Dolan SM, Tough SC. Cumulative psychosocial stress, coping resources, and preterm birth. Arch Womens Ment Health. 2014;17(6):559–68.
12. Challis J, Matthews S, Van Meir C, Ramirez M. Current topic: the placental corticotrophin-releasing hormone-adrenocorticotrophin axis. Placenta. 1995;16(6):481–502.
13. Goldenberg RL, Culhane JF, Iams JD, Romero R. Epidemiology and causes of preterm birth. Lancet. 2008;371(9606):75–84.
14. McCormick MC, Litt JS, Smith VC, Zupancic JA. Prematurity: an overview and public health implications. Annu Rev Public Health. 2011;32:367–79.
15. Kramer MS, Demissie K, Yang H, Platt RW, Sauvé R, Liston R, et al. The contribution of mild and moderate preterm birth to infant mortality. JAMA. 2000;284(7):843–9.
16. Martin JA, Kirmeyer S, Osterman M, Shepherd RA. Born a bit too early: recent trends in "late preterm" births. NCHS Data Brief. 2009;24:1–8.
17. Richards JL, Kramer MS, Deb-Rinker P, Rouleau J, Mortensen L, Gissler M, et al. Temporal trends in late preterm and early term birth rates in 6 high-income countries in North America and Europe and association with clinician-initiated obstetric interventions. JAMA. 2016;316(4):410–9.

18. Bilgin A, Wolke D. Maternal sensitivity in parenting preterm children: a meta-analysis. Pediatrics. 2015;136:1–17.
19. Feldman R, Rosenthal Z, Eidelman AI. Maternal-preterm skin-to-skin contact enhances child physiologic organization and cognitive control across the first 10 years of life. Biol Psychiatry. 2014;75(1):56–64.
20. Anderson C, Cacola P. Implications of preterm birth for maternal mental health and infant development. MCN Am J Matern Child Nurs. 2017;42(2):108–14.
21. Fisk NM, Glover V. Association between maternal anxiety in pregnancy and increased uterine artery resistance index: cohort based study. BMJ. 1999;318(7177):153–7.
22. Weaver IC, Cervoni N, Champagne FA, D'Alessio AC, Sharma S, Seckl JR, et al. Epigenetic programming by maternal behavior. Nat Neurosci. 2004;7(8):847–54.
23. Glover V. Prenatal stress and its effects on the fetus and the child: possible underlying biological mechanisms. Adv Neurobiol. 2015;10:269–83.
24. Glover V. Maternal depression, anxiety and stress during pregnancy and child outcome; what needs to be done. Best Pract Res Clin Obstet Gynaecol. 2014;28(1):25–35.
25. Jaekel J, Wolke D, Chernova J. Mother and child behaviour in very preterm and term dyads at 6 and 8 years. Dev Med Child Neurol. 2012;54(8):716–23.
26. Beckwith L, Rodning C. Dyadic processes between mothers and preterm infants: Development at ages 2 to 5 years. Infant Ment Health J. 1996;17(4):322–33.
27. Meyer EC, Coll CTG, Seifer R, Ramos A, Kilis E, Oh W. Psychological distress in mothers of preterm infants. J Dev Behav Pediatr. 1995;16(6):412–7.
28. Pierrehumbert B, Brisch K, Nicole A, Fava-Vizziello G, Wolke D. The processes of parenting and attachment with premature infants: implications for intervention. Infant Mental Health J. 2000: Michigan ASSN Infant Mental Health Michigan State Univ Dept Psychology, East Lansing, MI, USA
29. Muller-Nix C, Forcada-Guex M, Pierrehumbert B, Jaunin L, Borghini A, Ansermet F. Prematurity, maternal stress and mother–child interactions. Early Hum Dev. 2004;79(2): 145–58.
30. Landry SH, Smith KE, Swank PR. Responsive parenting: establishing early foundations for social, communication, and independent problem-solving skills. DP. 2006;42(4):627.
31. Lyons-Ruth K, Bureau J-F, Holmes B, Easterbrooks A, Brooks NH. Borderline symptoms and suicidality/self-injury in late adolescence: prospectively observed relationship correlates in infancy and childhood. Psychiatry Res. 2013;206(2):273–81.
32. Jaekel J, Pluess M, Belsky J, Wolke D. Effects of maternal sensitivity on low birth weight children's academic achievement: a test of differential susceptibility versus diathesis stress. J Child Psychol Psychiatry. 2015;56(6):693–701.
33. Engle WA, Tomashek KM, Wallman C. "Late-preterm" infants: a population at risk. Pediatrics. 2007;120(6):1390–401.
34. Voegtline KM, Stifter CA, Investigators FLP. Late-preterm birth, maternal symptomatology, and infant negativity. Infant Behav Dev. 2010;33(4):545–54.
35. Holditch-Davis D, Schwartz T, Black B, Scher M. Correlates of mother–premature infant interactions. Res Nurs Health. 2007;30(3):333–46.
36. Braungart-Rieker JM, Garwood MM, Powers BP, Wang X. Parental sensitivity, infant affect, and affect regulation: predictors of later attachment. Child Dev. 2001;72(1):252–70.
37. Amir M, Horesh N, Lin-Stein T. Infertility and adjustment in women: the effects of attachment style and social support. J Clin Psychol Med Settings. 1999;6(4):463–79.
38. Bowlby J. Attachment and loss: separation. 2nd ed. New York, NY: Basic Books; 1973.
39. Stuart S, Robertson M. Interpersonal psychotherapy 2E a clinician's guide. Boca Raton, FL: CRC Press; 2012.
40. Collins NL. Working models of attachment: Implications for explanation, emotion, and behavior. JPSP. 1996;71(4):810.
41. Simpson JA, Rholes WS. Adult attachment, stress, and romantic relationships. Curr Opin Psychol. 2017;13:19–24.

42. Dunkel-Schetter C, Tanner L. Anxiety, depression and stress in pregnancy: implications for mothers, children, research, and practice. Curr Opin Psychiatry. 2012;25(2):141.
43. Lou HC, Hansen D, Nordentoft M, Pryds O, Jensen F, Nim J, et al. Prenatal stressors of human life affect fetal brain development. Dev Med Child Neurol. 1994;36(9): 826–32.
44. Chaplin TM, Aldao A. Gender differences in emotion expression in children: a meta-analytic review. Psychol Bull. 2013;139(4):735–65.
45. Aarnoudse-Moens CSH, Weisglas-Kuperus N, van Goudoever JB, Oosterlaan J. Meta-analysis of neurobehavioral outcomes in very preterm and/or very low birth weight children. Pediatrics. 2009;124(2):717–28.
46. Wenzel A, Stuart SC. Anxiety in childbearing women: diagnosis and treatment. Washington, DC: American Psychological Association; 2011.
47. Davies J, Slade P, Wright I, Stewart P. Posttraumatic stress symptoms following childbirth and mothers' perceptions of their infants. Infant Ment Health J. 2008;29(6):537–54.
48. Ferber SG, Feldman R. Delivery pain and the development of mother—infant interaction. Infancy. 2005;8(1):43–62.
49. Grant KA, McMahon C, Austin MP. Maternal anxiety during the transition to parenthood: a prospective study. J Affect Disord. 2008;108(1–2):101–11.
50. Hildingsson I, Nilsson C, Karlström A, Lundgren I. A longitudinal survey of childbirth-related fear and associated factors. J Obstet Gynecol Neonatal Nurs. 2011;40(5):532–43.
51. Giallo R, Woolhouse H, Gartland D, Hiscock H, Brown S. The emotional–behavioural functioning of children exposed to maternal depressive symptoms across pregnancy and early childhood: a prospective Australian pregnancy cohort study. Eur Child Adolesc Psychiatry. 2015;24(10):1233–44.
52. van der Waerden J, Galera C, Saurel-Cubizolles MJ, Sutter-Dallay AL, Melchior M. Predictors of persistent maternal depression trajectories in early childhood: results from the EDEN mother-child cohort study in France. Psychol Med. 2015;45(9):1999–2012.
53. Kingston D, Tough S. Prenatal and postnatal maternal mental health and school-age child development: a systematic review. Matern Child Health J. 2014;18(7):1728–41.
54. Nilsson C, Lundgren I, Karlström A, Hildingsson I. Self reported fear of childbirth and its association with women's birth experience and mode of delivery: a longitudinal population-based study. Women Birth. 2012;25(3):114–21.
55. Waldenström U, Hildingsson I, Ryding E-L. Antenatal fear of childbirth and its association with subsequent caesarean section and experience of childbirth. BJOG. 2006;113(6):638–46.
56. Mughal MK, Ginn CS, Magill-Evans J, Benzies KM. Parenting stress and development of late preterm infants at 4 months corrected age. Res Nurs Health. 2017;40(5):414–23.
57. Baker BJ. Understanding mothers of late preterm infants. Richmond, VA: Virginia Commonwealth University; 2011.
58. Røsand G-MB, Slinning K, Eberhard-Gran M, Røysamb E, Tambs K. Partner relationship satisfaction and maternal emotional distress in early pregnancy. BMC Public Health. 2011;11(1):161.
59. Letourneau NL, Dennis C-L, Benzies K, Duffett-Leger L, Stewart M, Tryphonopoulos PD, et al. Postpartum depression is a family affair: addressing the impact on mothers, fathers, and children. Issues Ment Health Nurs. 2012;33(7):445–57.
60. Meighan M, Davis MW, Thomas SP, Droppleman PG. Living with postpartum depression: the father's experience. MCN Am J Matern Child Nurs. 1999;24(4):202–8.
61. Sayers SL, Kohn CS, Fresco DM, Bellack AS, Sarwer DB. Marital cognitions and depression in the context of marital discord. Cognit Ther Res. 2001;25(6):713–32.
62. Paulson JF, Bazemore SD. Prenatal and postpartum depression in fathers and its association with maternal depression: a meta-analysis. JAMA. 2010;303(19):1961–9.
63. Lee TY, Miles MS, Holditch-Davis D. Fathers' support to mothers of medically fragile infants. J Obstet Gynecol Neonatal Nurs. 2006;35(1):46–55.
64. Fox SE, Levitt P, Nelson CA III. How the timing and quality of early experiences influence the development of brain architecture. Child Dev. 2010;81(1):28–40.

65. Ulrich-Lai YM, Herman JP. Neural regulation of endocrine and autonomic stress responses. Nat Rev Neurosci. 2009;10(6):397.
66. Saisto T, Halmesmäki E. Fear of childbirth: a neglected dilemma. Acta Obstet Gynecol Scand. 2003;82(3):201–8.
67. American Psychiatric Association. Diagnostic and statistical manual of mental disorders (DSM-5®). Washington, DC: American Psychiatric Pub; 2013.
68. Kleiman K, Wenzel A. Dropping the baby and other scary thoughts: breaking the cycle of unwanted thoughts in motherhood. London: Routledge; 2011.
69. Matthey S, Ross-Hamid C. The validity of DSM symptoms for depression and anxiety disorders during pregnancy. J Affect Disord. 2011;133(3):546–52.
70. Huizink AC, Mulder EJ, de Medina PGR, Visser GH, Buitelaar JK. Is pregnancy anxiety a distinctive syndrome? Early Hum Dev. 2004;79(2):81–91.
71. Lang AJ, Sorrell JT, Rodgers CS, Lebeck MM. Anxiety sensitivity as a predictor of labor pain. Eur J Pain. 2006;10(3):263.
72. White T, Matthey S, Boyd K, Barnett B. Postnatal depression and post-traumatic stress after childbirth: prevalence, course and co-occurrence. J Reprod Infant Psychol. 2006;24(02):107–20.
73. Kelly RH, Russo J, Katon W. Somatic complaints among pregnant women cared for in obstetrics: normal pregnancy or depressive and anxiety symptom amplification revisited? Gen Hosp Psychiatry. 2001;23(3):107–13.
74. Austin MP, Priest SR. Clinical issues in perinatal mental health: new developments in the detection and treatment of perinatal mood and anxiety disorders. Acta Psychiatr Scand. 2005;112(2):97–104.
75. Lee AM, Lam SK, Lau SMSM, Chong CSY, Chui HW, Fong DYT. Prevalence, course, and risk factors for antenatal anxiety and depression. Obstet Gynecol. 2007;110(5):1102–12.
76. Kuo C, Chen G, Yang M, Lo H, Tsai Y. Biphasic changes in autonomic nervous activity during pregnancy. Br J Anaesth. 2000;84(3):323–9.
77. Yonkers KA, Smith MV, Lin H, Howell HB, Shao L, Rosenheck RA. Depression screening of perinatal women: an evaluation of the healthy start depression initiative. Psychiatr Serv. 2009;60(3):322–8.
78. De Jesus Silva MM, Peres-Rocha-Carvalho-Leite E, Alves-Nogueira D, Clapis MJ. Depression in pregnancy. Prevalence and associated factors. Invest Educ Enferm. 2016;34(2):342–50.
79. Smith KF, Huber LRB, Issel LM, Warren-Findlow J. The association between maternal depression during pregnancy and adverse birth outcomes: a retrospective cohort study of PRAMS participants. J Community Health. 2015;40(5):984–92.
80. Manikkam L, Burns JK. Antenatal depression and its risk factors: an urban prevalence study in KwaZulu-Natal. S Afr Med J. 2012;102(12):940–4.
81. World Health Organization. Thinking healthy: a manual for psychosocial management of perinatal depression, WHO generic field-trial version 1.0, 2015. Geneva: WHO; 2015.
82. NICE. Antenatal and postnatal mental health: clinical management and service guidance (CG192). London: NICE – National Institute for Health and Care Excellence; 2014.
83. Somerville S, Dedman K, Hagan R, Oxnam E, Wettinger M, Byrne S, et al. The perinatal anxiety screening scale: development and preliminary validation. Arch Womens Ment Health. 2014;17(5):443–54.
84. Somerville S, Byrne SL, Dedman K, Hagan R, Coo S, Oxnam E, et al. Detecting the severity of perinatal anxiety with the Perinatal Anxiety Screening Scale (PASS). J Affect Disord. 2015;186:18–25.
85. Bayrampour H, McDonald S, Tough S. Risk factors of transient and persistent anxiety during pregnancy. Midwifery. 2015;31(6):582–9.
86. Zigmond AS, Snaith RP. The hospital anxiety and depression scale. Acta Psychiatr Scand. 1983;67(6):361–70.
87. Spielberger CD, Gorsuch RL, Lushene R, Vagg PR, Jacobs G. State-trait anxiety inventory for adults. Menlo Park, CA: Mind Garden; 1983.
88. Beck A, Steer R. Beck anxiety inventory manual. San Antonio, TX: The Psychological Corporation; 1993.

89. Levin JS. The factor structure of the pregnancy anxiety scale. J Health Soc Behav. 1991;32:368–81.
90. Wadhwa PD, Sandman CA, Porto M, Dunkel-Schetter C, Garite TJ. The association between prenatal stress and infant birth weight and gestational age at birth: a prospective investigation. Am J Obstet Gynecol. 1993;169(4):858–65.
91. Van den Bergh B. The influence of maternal emotions during pregnancy on fetal and neonatal behavior. Pre Perinat Psychol J. 1990;5(2):119–30.
92. Rwakarema M, Premji SS, Nyanza EC, Riziki P, Palacios-Derflingher L. Antenatal depression is associated with pregnancy-related anxiety, partner relations, and wealth in women in Northern Tanzania: a cross-sectional study. BMC Womens Health. 2015;15(1):68.
93. Rini CK, Dunkel-Schetter C, Wadhwa PD, Sandman CA. Psychological adaptation and birth outcomes: the role of personal resources, stress, and sociocultural context in pregnancy. Health Psychol. 1999;18(4):333–45.
94. Cox JL, Holden JM, Sagovsky R. Detection of postnatal depression. Development of the 10-item Edinburgh Postnatal Depression Scale. Br J Psychiatry. 1987;150:782–6.
95. Murray D, Cox JL. Screening for depression during pregnancy with the Edinburgh Depression Scale (EDDS). J Reprod Infant Psychol. 1990;8(2):99–107.
96. Bambridge GA, Shaw EJ, Ishak M, Clarke SD, Baker C. Perinatal mental health: how to ask and how to help. Obstet Gynaecol. 2017;19(2):147–53.
97. Howard LM, Molyneaux E, Dennis C-L, Rochat T, Stein A, Milgrom J. Non-psychotic mental disorders in the perinatal period. Lancet. 2014;384(9956):1775–88.
98. Dennis CL, Chung-Lee L. Postpartum depression help-seeking barriers and maternal treatment preferences: a qualitative systematic review. Birth. 2006;33(4):323–31.
99. Schwarzer R, Knoll N. Functional roles of social support within the stress and coping process: a theoretical and empirical overview. Int J Psychol. 2007;42(4):243–52.
100. Nurullah AS. Received and provided social support: a review of current evidence and future directions. Am J Health Stud. 2012;27(3):173–88.
101. Champion L. Social relationships and social roles. Clin Psychol Psychother. 2012;19(2):113–23.
102. Cutrona CE, Russell DW. Autonomy promotion, responsiveness, and emotion regulation promote effective social support in times of stress. Curr Opin Psychol. 2017;13:126–30.
103. Cohen S, McKay G. Social support, stress and the buffering hypothesis: a theoretical analysis. Handb Psychol Health. 1984;4:253–67.
104. Ozturk Z, Olmez E, Gurpinar T, Gok S, Vural K. Safety of psychotropic medications in pregnancy: an observational cohort study. Bull Clin Psychopharmacol. 2016;26(3):229–37.

What Do I Need to Know About the Father of a Late Preterm Infant so I Can Support Him in the Postpartum Period?

4

Shahirose Sadrudin Premji and Gianella Santos Pana

4.1 Background

Around the globe there is a commitment to maternal, newborn, and child health care in hopes of reducing neonatal and child mortality. Fathers remain at the periphery of these initiatives both during pregnancy and postpartum [1]. Animal and emerging human studies suggest that the transition to fatherhood is marked by adaptive changes in the brain and biological responses of hormones such as oxytocin, testosterone, and prolactin that promote (a) nurturing and supportive behaviors toward mothers and infants, (b) paternal attachment with infant through play, and (c) altered interactions and sexual behavior (i.e., less abuse, violence, risk taking behaviors, and sexual intercourse) [1–8]. The brain's architecture and function is influenced by life experiences including the birth of an infant between $34^{0/7}$ gestational weeks and $36^{6/7}$ gestational weeks (i.e., late preterm infant (LPI)), stress, worries or fears, and adverse early life experiences [9]. Paternal depression, both during the first trimester and after pregnancy (3–9 months), has been reported in 8–10% of men [10, 11] and influences maternal depression [11] and paternal-infant interaction [12]. Paternal mental health and paternal-infant interactions impact emotional and behavioral development of the child in unique ways [13, 14] which has significant implications for LPIs as they are at a higher risk of neurodevelopmental impairments [15, 16]. In this chapter we explore how fathers respond to the birth of their LPI, adjust to parenthood, and interact with their LPI by undertaking a critical and narrative review [17, 18] of all available literature examining fathers of LPIs. What we learn about fathers of LPIs will

S. S. Premji (✉)
School of Nursing, Faculty of Health, York University, Toronto, ON, Canada
e-mail: premjis@yorku.ca

G. S. Pana
Birth Doula, Chavah Childbirth Services Inc., Calgary, AB, Canada

Faculty of Nursing, University of Calgary, Calgary, AB, Canada
e-mail: gspana@ucalgary.ca

© Springer International Publishing AG, part of Springer Nature 2019
S. S. Premji (ed.), *Late Preterm Infants*, https://doi.org/10.1007/978-3-319-94352-7_4

inform how we can include fathers in maternal, newborn, and child care and support them along the continuum of pregnancy (i.e., prenatal and postnatal period).

4.2   Type of Review

In general, the body of literature on fathers and their infants is limited and varies with respect to types of studies and scope (i.e., broad); thus a traditional systematic methodology is not appropriate [17]. Our review approach is critical in its emphasis on relevance and involves an extensive search of literature from diverse sources to determine what we know about fathers of LPIs that will guide our practice [18]. We have used a narrative style in which themes identified through interpretive synthesis of the available literature, regardless of the research approach, are shared in the results [17]. The goal is not to assess the quality of the studies and generate theory but through subjective interpretation identify key areas of emphasis related to the care of fathers with LPIs [17, 18].

4.3   Search Strategy

Five electronic databases—Medline (1946 to March 2018), Embase (1974 to March 2018), Cochrane Central Register of Controlled Trials (1972 to February 2018), PsycINFO (1806 to March 2018), and CINAHL (1982 to March 2018)—were searched. Search terms comprised a combination of related terms describing both the late preterm infant and fathers. Key terms for late preterm included late preterm, late premature, near(ly) term, moderate(ly) preterm, and moderate(ly) premature. Key terms for infant included infant, newborn, neonate, baby, babies, and preemie(s). Key terms for father included father, dad, paternal, men, male parent, and husband. There were no limits (publication type, study type, time, etc.) applied on the search for paternal literature. A total of 104 records were identified initially which yielded 51 unique records. One reviewer (SP) screened the title and abstracts for relevance and then scrutinized the full texts of the remaining records according to the inclusion criteria: (a) focus on fathers, (b) in relation to late preterm infants defined as those born between $34^{0/7}$ weeks' gestational age and $36^{6/7}$ weeks' gestational age, and (c) any phenomena (e.g., experience of fatherhood, mental health, parent-infant interaction). Although seven full-text records were relevant, two records [19, 20] were identical, being published as abstract [19] and full-text article [20]. Three records [20–22] are part of the same study but given their unique contributions have been included as separate articles. Thus, six articles [20–25] were included in this critical and narrative review (see Fig. 4.1 "Flow diagram of studies"). The reference list of the six included articles was reviewed, and no additional literature was identified. We have included theoretical and research literature on fathers and infants where appropriate to extend our understanding of the themes identified, namely, father's influence on neurodevelopment of LPI, father-infant interaction, and paternal emotional distress.

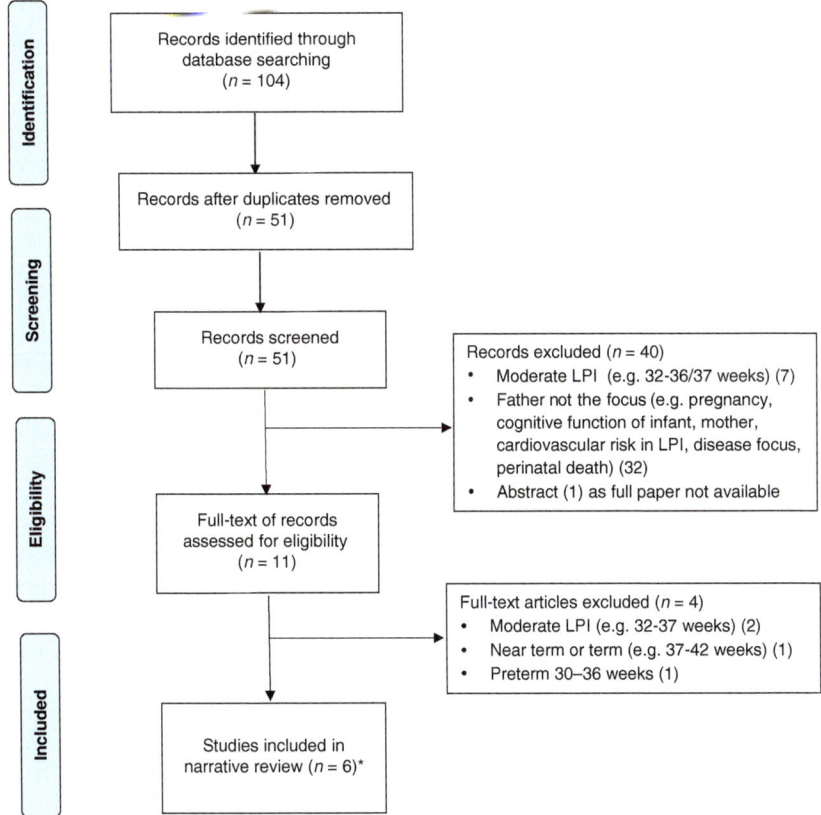

* Abstract published in conference proceedings was the same as full-text article published under a different title.

Fig. 4.1 Flow diagram of studies

4.4   Results

4.4.1   Father's Influence on Neurodevelopment of LPI

LPIs, by arriving 4–6 weeks early, may be more sensitive, in differing or varied ways, to environmental effects that are both beneficial and harmful for them [24, 26]. If indeed this is true, then LPIs have the "plasticity factor" (i.e., differential susceptibility), and we have an opportunity to improve their neurodevelopmental outcomes through paternal caregiving environments [24]. However, social, cognitive, and motor skills of LPIs were not affected by paternal emotional distress or paternal quality of attachment, suggesting there is limited evidence of plasticity factor [24]. Alternately, for very preterm infants, fathers' emotional distress did, however, impact very preterm infants' cognitive and socioemotional development [24]. The authors [24] surmise that their data, to some extent, support an alternate theory of diathesis-stress whereby infants born earlier and exposed to the same environmental factors as those born later will have worse outcomes [27]. Moreover, poor paternal caregiving environment will impact those who are more vulnerable [28]. Thus, very preterm infants may be more susceptible to poor paternal caregiving environment than late preterm infants.

Language development depends on reciprocal (i.e., two sided) vocalizations or conversation between parent and child [29]. Parent talk with preterm infants in the neonatal intensive care unit promotes cognitive development at 7 and 18 months corrected age [30]. In a study where 55% of the sample were late preterm infants, fathers not only had strikingly less verbal interaction with their infants, they responded less frequently to their infant's vocalization from birth through 7 months when compared to mothers [23]. In the first month of life, infants preferentially respond to their mother's voice [23]. Father's appeared to be more responsive to vocalization of boys although findings were not statistically significant [23]. In two-parent families with low-income and residing in rural communities in United States, fathers' vocal interactions predicted communication development and language development at 15 months and 36 months of age, respectively [31].

4.4.2 Father–Infant Interaction

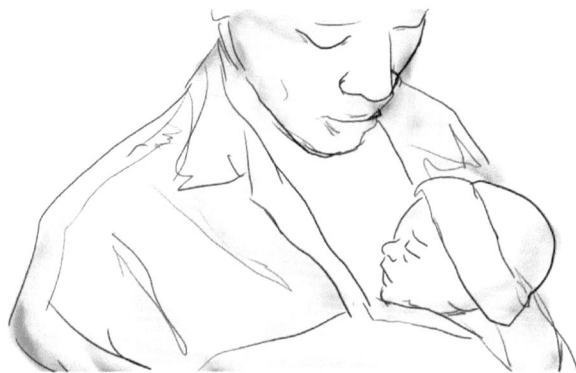

Skin-to-skin care is one component of Kangaroo Mother Care [25]. Kangaroo Mother Care also includes breastfeeding (ideally exclusive breastfeeding), early discharge when physiologically stable, feeding, and appropriate follow-up visits until gaining weight and thriving [32]. Although fathers practice skin-to-skin care with their LPIs during the first and second day of life, it is comparably less than half the time LPIs spend skin-to-skin with their mother [25]. The infants' duration of skin-to-skin with father during the first day after birth, rather than the mother, was associated with exclusive breastfeeding at discharge [25]. Fathers' duration of time in skin-to-skin contact with the LPI decreased from day 1 to day 2 of life. Duration of time was associated with time of birth (more at night), infant's gender (more with boys), and mode of delivery (more if born by caesarean section) during the first day after birth and infant's birth weight (more if low birth weight), time point of birth (more if born at night), parity (first baby), and if supplemental feeding (shorter time SSC) during the second day after birth [25].

In a randomized controlled trial, fathers were video recorded in a structured play interaction when their infant was 4 months of age [21]. In the intervention group the recording was reviewed immediately with father while reinforcing strengths and providing one or two suggestions to encourage language development while in the comparison group the video was not reviewed; however information was provided about age-appropriate play. Those receiving four visits (4, 5, 6, 7, and 8 months) had more optimal father-infant interactions than fathers in the comparison group [21]. The intervention, however, did not reduce parenting stress nor change fathers perceptions of the LPIs temperament and behavior (i.e., child domain) [21]. A subsample of these fathers (see Table 4.1 for details of the study) enrolled in a qualitative study at 8 months corrected age explained that they felt overwhelmed at times as fathering was the "biggest job ever" … bigger than they ever imagined ([20], p. 81). Although things got easier, they were preoccupied with their LPIs developmental progress, ensuring the safety of their LPI, financial security, and balancing the demands of work and home ([20], p. 81–82).

4.4.3 Paternal Emotional Distress

Bronfenbrenner's ecological model theorizes that the infant's immediate environment or microsystem, both physical and social, can negatively affect infant development [33]. Parenting stress, an aspect of this immediate environment, is multidimensional being influenced by parent characteristics, infant characteristics and needs, situational factors, parental emotional state (i.e., anxiety, depression), confidence in care, and coping [34–36]. As such, parenting stress can influence parent-infant interactions whereby the parent affects the infant and infant affects the parent both in ways that negatively affects the infant's development [33]. At 4 months corrected age, fathers of LPIs report less stress when compared with mothers of LPIs with respect to the parent domain [22]. Moreover, fathers' stress was not correlated to infant development as measured by various domains on Ages & Stages Questionnaire (2nd edition) (e.g., communication, personal-social domains) [22]. At 8 months corrected age, a subsample of fathers enrolled in the same study used words like "awesome," "fulfilling," "very rewarding," "a whole lot of fun, and a lot of work," and the "best thing ever" in response to questions like "How has fathering been going for you?," "What are your joys?," and "What are your concerns?" ([22], p. 80–81). With respect to the child domain, concerns related to their LPI's developmental progress include weight gain, vocalizing, walking, and

Table 4.1 Overview of included studies

Study and country	Objective/purpose	Type of study and design	Sample	Data collection method	Major findings with focus on fathers	Comments
Hadfield et al. [24] Ireland	"Test whether the effects of mothers' and fathers' emotional distress and quality of attachment on child outcomes differed by level of prematurity. Hypothesis: early and late preterm status would be associated with less positive social, cognitive, and mother skills outcomes" (p. 28).	Quantitative: growing up in Ireland National Infant Cohort Study: secondary analysis with first two waves. Wave 1 data (September 2008 to April 2009) at 9-month-old infants and wave 2 data (December 2010 to July 2011) after child's 3rd birthday.	National representative sample from Child Benefit Register Very preterm (≤33 weeks) = 231; late preterm (34–36 weeks) = 513; full-term (≥37 weeks) = 10,390; fathers = 9998.	*Fathers* Emotional distress measures: 18-item Parental Stress Scale; 8-item Center for Epidemiological Studies Depression Scale (CES-D) (p. 31); Quality of Attachment: 5-item version Quality of Attachment subscale which asked about feelings toward infant and them as parent (p. 31). *Infants* Outcomes at 3 years of age—socio-emotional skills, Strengths and Difficulties Questionnaire; Cognitive Development, Picture Similarities and Naming Vocabulary subscales; motor skills, tasks stand on one leg, throw a ball overhand, copy a vertical line, and use a pincer grip (1 point per task with total 0 to 4) (p. 32).	When compared with full-term infants, being born late preterm was associated with poorer cognitive functioning only. Social, cognitive, and motor skills of late preterm infants are not affected by paternal caregiving variables. Late preterm infants are not more vulnerable to environmental influences (i.e., no support for plasticity factor). Note: In the case of very preterm infants, however, fathers' emotional distress impacted their cognitive and socioemotional development.	Extracted data relevant to fathers only. Focusing on variables relevant to fathers of LPI. Level of prematurity as covariate.

Nyqvist et al. [25] Sweden	"to investigate the duration of healthy late preterm infants' SSC [skin-to-skin contact] with the mother and father, respectively, during the first 48 h after birth and its associations with breastfeeding, clinical and demographic variables" (p. 3).	Quantitative: Observational cohort study.	64 healthy late preterm infants. Inclusion criteria: Swedish-speaking parents, cared for in family rooms at postnatal ward, Uppsala University Hospital. Healthy = no neonatal intensive care unit, no morbidities (e.g., respiratory, hypoglycemia, infection, or feeding).	Parental diary with chart for each day to record timing and duration of SSC by mother, father, or others, duration of breastfeeding, supplementary feedings. Data on first 48 h. Demographic (e.g., age, sex, weight, etc.) and clinical variables (e.g., mode of delivery, fetal asphyxia, etc.).	Fathers spend less than half the time mothers do giving SSC. First day: time fathers spend giving SSC was associated with time of birth (more at night), infant's gender (more with boys), and mode of delivery (more if born by caesarean section). Second day: time fathers spend giving SSC was associate infant's birth weight (more if low birth weight), time point of birth (more if born at night), parity (first baby), and if supplemental feeding (shorter time SSC). "Exclusive breastfeeding at discharge was significantly associated with infants' duration of SSC with fathers during the first day after birth, whereas no associations were found with mothers"(p. 13).	Highlight da.a related to fathers only.

(continued)

Table 4.1 (continued)

Study and country	Objective/purpose	Type of study and design	Sample	Data collection method	Major findings with focus on fathers	Comments
Mughal et al. [22] Canada	"to examine the relationships between parenting stress in mothers and fathers who were co-parenting their late preterm infants and child development at 4 months corrected age" (p. 415).	Quantitative: Cross-sectional study. Reporting data on 108 of 111 fathers enrolled in the larger study conducted between December 2008 and June 2011.	108 fathers of late preterm infants ($34^{0/7}$–$36^{6/7}$ weeks of gestation) who had complete questionnaire data. Inclusion criteria: first-time, biological father of a healthy, singleton, late preterm infant; English-speaking in at least 50% of interactions with infant; age 18 years or older; cohabiting with infant's other biological parent; and living within 100 km of the university.	*Fathers* Paternal stress at infant's corrected age of 4 months: Parenting Stress Index–third edition (PSI-3)—120-item self-reported measure of stress associated with parenting children from 1 month to 12 years (p. 416). *Infants* Development at infant's corrected age of 4 months: Ages & Stages Questionnaire–second edition (ASQ-2)—37-item parent-reported development screener to capture risk of delay in children ages 4–60 months. In this study, the ASQ-2 was completed by mothers because in most cases mothers were the primary caregivers (p. 416).	Fathers had significantly less stress co-parenting their LPIs than mothers. No correlations were found between paternal stress and infant development at 4 months.	Extracted data relevant to fathers only.

Benzies et al. [20] Canada	"to explore fathers' experiences and their perceptions of the intervention" (p. 80).	Qualitative: Semi-structured qualitative interview. Reporting data on 85 of 111 fathers enrolled in the larger study conducted between December 2008 and June 2011.	85 fathers late preterm infants (34⁰ᐟ⁷–36⁶ᐟ⁷ weeks of gestation) from one center. Inclusion criteria: first-time, biological father of a healthy, singleton, late preterm infant; English-speaking in at least 50% of interactions with infant; age 18 years or older; cohabiting with infant's other biological parent; and living within 100 km of the university.	"At the 8-month outcome visit, the home visitor captured fathers' experiences using a semi-structured qualitative interview: fathers were encouraged to speak freely about topics of interest to them" (p. 80).	The joys of fatherhood: fathers talked about instances of spending time with the baby, watching the baby grow and learn, and the baby being excited to see dad. The challenges of fatherhood: fathers were concerned about keeping the baby safe, the baby lagging in development, and their ability to be a good father, provide for their family, and balance demands of home and work. Fatherhood as an opportunity for personal growth: "fathers described the transition to fatherhood as better than they expected and revealed how fatherhood made a huge difference in their lives" (p. 82). Fathers recommend easily accessible information and resources that improved their confidence, knowledge, and skills as a father as well as meet a variety of needs.	Highlight data related to father's experience with their infant.

(continued)

Table 4.1 (continued)

Study and country	Objective/purpose	Type of study and design	Sample	Data collection method	Major findings with focus on fathers	Comments
Johnson et al. [23] United States	Assess infant's language environment in the first months of life, and determine if there are differences based on adult (i.e., mother versus father) and gender (i.e., infant male versus female) Hypotheses: (1) infants will be exposed to female speech more so than male speech, (2) fathers will have less reciprocal vocalizations with infants when compared to mothers, and (3) there will be gender differences with female infants having more vocalizations and conversational exchanges (p. e1604).	Quantitative: Prospective cohort study. Reporting data on 33 of 81 infants enrolled in the larger study conducted between February 2010 and May 2012. Note: study infants differed from those not included in the study.	Total 33 infants: 18 healthy late preterm infants ($34^{0/7}$ to $36^{6/7}$ weeks) and 15 term infants ($37^{0/7}$ to $41^{6/7}$) recruited during birth hospitalization. Inclusion criteria: medically stable, no congenital anomalies, comorbidities or hearing impairment, living in a two-parent home, and 10 h full-length recordings at birth, 44 weeks postmenstrual age, and 7 months of age.	Digital language processors worn by each infant for 16 continuous hours of recording at birth hospital, 44 weeks postmenstrual age, and 7 months. Language environment analysis system (LENA) used to monitor speech and language environment and report: infant vocalization counts, adult word counts, and conversational turn counts.	In hospital NICU: less speech Rooming-in: more speech After discharge NICU infants: meaningful speech increased Normal newborn: decreased Overall increase in language exposure over time. Hypotheses: (1) supported as infants have more female adult speech exposure from birth through 7 months, (2) supported as females respond more frequently than males to their infants' vocalization from birth through 7 months. Infants show a preference to vocal responses of their mothers in the first month of life, and (3) at birth and 44 weeks gestation, mothers respond preferentially to girls than boys. Data suggests trend that fathers preferentially respond to boys at 44 weeks postmenstrual age and 7 months.	Did not compare late preterm infants and term infants.

| Benzies et al. [21] Canada | "to evaluate the effect of an intervention for fathers of late preterm infants, seeking to optimize one aspect of the infant's environment" (p. 334) Hypothesis: "compared with fathers of late preterm infants who received information only, fathers who received the video self-modeling with feedback intervention would have better father-infant interaction skills when the child was 8 months old (corrected age)" (p. 336). | Quantitative: Randomized controlled trial with a dose optimization study. | Total 111 fathers: two-dose intervention group = 46; four-dose intervention group = 23; comparison group = 42. Inclusion criteria: first-time, biological father of a healthy, singleton, late preterm infant ($34^{0/7}$–$36^{6/7}$ weeks of gestation); English-speaking in at least 50% of interactions with infant; age 18 years or older; cohabiting with infant's other biological parent; and living within 100 km of the university. | Father-infant interactions were assessed using the Parent Child Interaction Teaching Scale (PCITS) protocol and video recorded. Intervention group: after a structured play interaction, the father and home visitor would immediately review the video. The home visitor reinforced the fathers' strengths and made one or two suggestions. The two-visit intervention group received home visits at the infant's corrected age of 4, 6, and 8 months; the four-visit group received visits at age 4, 5, 6, 7, and 8 months. Comparison group: the video was not viewed, and home visitors discussed general information about age-appropriate play. The comparison group received home visits at age 4 and 8 months. At 4 months corrected age, a questionnaire package (PSI-3 & WPL-R) was mailed to the family. PSI-3: 120-item self-report instrument which measures parenting stress and perceptions of the child's temperament and behavior. WPL-R: 25-item self-report instrument which measures perceptions of parenting a young infant. | Hypothesis: supported as fathers who received the video self-modeling with feedback intervention over 4 visits had better father-infant interaction skills than the fathers who received information only. Fathers who received four home visits had improved father-infant interaction skills over time, while the skills of fathers in the comparison group worsened. The two home visits did not influence father-infant interaction skills. The intervention did not reduce parenting stress nor change fathers' perceptions of their LPIs' temperament and behavior or their perception of parenting their LPI. | Highlight data related to dose optimization interventions. |

general development ([22], p. 80–81). Of note, fathers did not link these concerns to their infants being born early (i.e., LPI). Self-confidence in caring for their LPI was an issue for these fathers—"Am I doing a good job and being a good parent?," "not knowing how to soothe her," and "don't know what the baby wants"—who believed this was the result of lack of knowledge and resources—"We don't know where to go for information to help us be better parents" ([20], p. 82). Fathers did, however, view fatherhood as surpassing their expectations in a positive way "better than I could have ever hoped it could be" and provided an opportunity for personal growth, for example, "changed everything including my feelings about life, the way I live my life, my expectations for the future – I am hopeful" ([20], p. 82). What is evident is that fathers of LPIs also feel excluded in maternal and newborn care as evident from statements like "Originally I wanted to be in the study because I felt excluded… parenting is stereotypically focused on mothers" and "there is a mindset that dads don't get involved with their babies until [age] 3 years" ([20], p. 82). Both fathers explained that we "need to change that" ([20], p. 82).

4.5   Discussion

Fathers of LPIs remain at the periphery in research as evident from the limited number of studies available for this review, the fact that they are secondary consideration in majority of these studies (i.e., secondary question or analysis of data), and fathers telling us this in a qualitative study. Our understanding about fathers of LPIs though limited does provide some important consideration for practice and research. The caregiving environment influences infants, particularly those who are vulnerable [28]. By being born 4–6 weeks earlier, LPIs' brain and organs continue to develop and are susceptible to environmental factors. Consequently, it makes sense to promote a positive paternal caregiving environment. The literature suggests there are two opportunities for this: skin-to-skin contact and reciprocal vocalization or conversation between father and their LPI.

Fathers appear to spend less time than mothers in skin-to-skin contact with their LPI, and the duration of time decreases in subsequent days after birth [25]. Health-care providers should provide ample opportunities and time to fathers to practice skin-to-skin with their LPI which may make fathers feel more included in maternal and newborn care. Moreover, enabling fathers to spend more time skin-to-skin with their LPI during the first day after birth may affect exclusive breastfeeding at discharge [25]. Health-care providers need to be mindful of contextual (e.g., mode of delivery) and sociocultural factors (e.g., gender preference) and intervene appropriately to influence fathers' uptake and duration of skin-to-skin in the postpartum period.

Bronfenbrenner's ecological model [33] and research studies in general support the assertion that paternal-infant interactions, especially reciprocal vocalizations or conversations between parent and infant, influence future cognitive, communication, and language development [29–31]. Some preliminary data suggests that fathers of LPIs have less verbal interactions with their infants and engage or respond infrequently to infant vocalization, especially if the infant is a girl [30]. Health-care providers need to promote father-infant interactions, with both boys and girls equally, and teach fathers the importance of these early interactions in promoting LPIs' neurodevelopmental outcomes. Skin-to-skin contact may be a starting point for fathers to interact verbally with their LPI and be responsive to vocalization of their LPI. Changing roles in society, with fathers spending more time in caregiving while women work to ensure financial stability in the household, makes it imperative for health-care providers to impart this knowledge to both parents. Innovation is required to increase knowledge and skills in achieving quality sensitive and response interactions with LPIs, as well as changing gendered care, that is, changing how fathers respond differently to male and female infants. The reciprocal nature of this relationship must be acknowledged as infants also respond preferentially to their mother's voice [23].

Finally, fathers respond differently to the birth of a LPI than mothers [22]. The literature is sparse in this area to understand the interrelationships between parent and infant characteristics, situation factors, parental emotional states (e.g., anxiety and depression), confidence in care, coping, and infant's development [33–36]. What is evident is that they may need different resources to cope with the birth of their LPI.

Conclusion
Fathers react and respond differently to LPIs when compared to mothers and need health-care providers to be attentive to them both during the postpartum period. Health-care providers should promote paternal-infant interactions right from birth and encourage fathers to talk with their infant and be responsive to their cues and vocalizations. Skin-to-skin contact is an ideal time for fathers to be attentive to facial expressions, sounds, or noises made by their LPI and socialize with their LPI (e.g., touch, talk, and music). Father's sensitivity and responsiveness to their LPIs will enable the LPI to reach their full developmental potential.

Take-Home Messages
- There is an opportunity to improve the neurodevelopmental outcomes of late preterm infants, and an under-researched yet fruitful area is through paternal caregiving environments which focus on father-infant interactions in the postpartum period.
- Health-care providers should provide opportunities for fathers to practice skin-to-skin contact and have reciprocal vocalization or conversation with their LPI since it can affect exclusive breastfeeding at discharge, promote neurodevelopment outcomes, and create an environment where fathers feel more included.
- It is imperative that health-care providers impart knowledge to both parents not only due to the health benefits for LPIs but also because of changes to societal roles and to acknowledge that mothers and fathers may need different resources to cope with the birth of their LPI.

References

1. Brown K. Rebuilding the triad: including fathers in maternal-child health. Pacific J Reprod Health. 2017;1(5):214–7. https://doi.org/10.18313/pjrh.2017.900.
2. Berg SJ, Wynne-Edwards KE. Changes in testosterone, cortisol, and estradiol, and estradiol levels in men becoming fathers. Mayo Clin Proc. 2001;76(6):582–92.
3. Carré JM, McCormick CM, Hariri AR. The social neuroendocrinology of human aggression. Psychoneuroendocrinology. 2011;36(7):935–44.
4. Edelstein RS, Chopik WJ, Saxbe DE, Wardecker BM, Moors AC, LaBelle OP. Prospective and dyadic associations between expectant parents' prenatal hormone changes and postpartum parenting outcomes. Dev Psychobiol. 2017;59(1):77–90.
5. Edelstein RS, Kean EL, Chopik WJ. Women with an avoidant attachment style show attenuated estradiol responses to emotionally intimate stimuli. Horm Behav. 2012;61(2):167–75.
6. Edelstein RS, Wardecker BM, Chopik WJ, Moors AC, Shipman EL, Lin NJ. Prenatal hormones in first-time expectant parents: Longitudinal changes and within-couple correlations. Am J Hum Biol. 2015;27(3):317–25.
7. Gettler LT, McDade TW, Agustin SS, Feranil AB, Kuzawa CW. Do testosterone declines during the transition to marriage and fatherhood relate to men's sexual behavior? Evidence from the Philippines. Horm Behav. 2013;64(5):755–63.
8. Wynne-Edwards KE. Hormonal changes in mammalian fathers. Horm Behav. 2001;40(2):139–45.
9. McEwen BS. Neurobiological and systemic effects of chronic stress. Chronic Stress. 2017;1:PMID:28856337. https://doi.org/10.1177/2470547017692328.
10. Cameron EE, Sedov ID, Tomfohr-Madsen LM. Prevalence of paternal depression in pregnancy and the postpartum: an updated meta-analysis. J Affect Disord. 2016;206:189–203. https://doi.org/10.1016/j.jad/2016.07.044.
11. Paulson JF, Bazemore SD. Prenatal and postpartum depression in fathers and its association with maternal depression: a meta-analysis. JAMA. 2010;303(19):1961–9. https://doi.org/10.1001/jama.2010.605.
12. Sethna V, Murray L, Edmondson O, Iles J, Ramchandani PG. Depression and playfulness in fathers and young infants: a matched design comparison study. J Affect Disord. 2018;229:364–70.
13. Luoma I, Puura K, Mäntymaa M, Latva R, Salmelin R, Tamminen T. Fathers' postnatal depressive and anxiety symptoms: an exploration of links with paternal, maternal, infant and family factors. Nord J Psychiatry. 2013;67(6):407–13. https://doi.org/10.3109/08039488.2012.752034. Epub 2013 Jan 3
14. Menashe-Grinberg A, Atzaba-Poria N. Mother-child and father-child play interaction: the importance of parental playfulness as a moderator of the links between parental behavior and child negativity. Infant Ment Health J. 2017;38(6):772–84. https://doi.org/10.1002/imhj.21678.
15. Munakata S, Okada T, Okahashi A, et al. Gray matter volumetric MRI differences late-preterm and term infants. Brain and Development. 2013;35:10–6.
16. Walsh JM, Doyle LW, Anderson PJ, Lee KJ, Cheong JL. Moderate and late preterm birth: effect on brain size and maturation at term-equivalent age. Radiology. 2014;273(1):232–40.
17. Dixon-Woods M, Cavers D, Agarwal S, Annandale E, Arthur A, Harvey J, et al. Conducting a critical interpretive synthesis of the literature on access to healthcare by vulnerable groups. BMC Med Res Methodol. 2006;6:35. https://doi.org/10.1186/1471-2288-6-35.
18. Grant MJ, Booth A. A typology of reviews: an analysis of 14 review types and associated methodologies. Health Inf Libr J. 2009;26(2):91–108. https://doi.org/10.1111/j.1471-1842.2009.00848.x.
19. Benzies K, Magill-Evans J. Giving voice to the experiences of first-time fathers of late preterm infants: a qualitative study. [Abstract]. Arch Dis Child. 2014;99(Supl 2):A1–A620.
20. Benzies K, Magill-Evans J. Through the eyes of a new dad: experiences of first-time fathers of late-preterm infants. Infant Ment Health J. 2015;36(1):78–87.

21. Benzies KM, Magill-Evans J, Kurilova J, Nettel-Aguirre A, Blahitka L, Lacaze-Masmonteil T. Effects of video-modeling on the interaction skills of first-time fathers of late preterm infants. Infants Young Children. 2013;26(4):333–48.

22. Mughal MKG, Carla S, Magill-Evans J, Benzies KM. Parenting stress and development of late preterm infants at 4 months corrected age. Res Nurs Health. 2017;40(5):414–23.

23. Johnson K, Caskey M, Rand K, Tucker R, Vohr B. Gender differences in adult-infant communication in the first months of life. Pediatrics. 2014;134(6):e1603–31610. https://doi.org/10.1542/peds.2013-4289.

24. Hadfield K, O'Brien F, Gerow A. Is the level of prematurity a risk/plasticity factor at three years of age? Infant Behav Dev. 2017;47:27–39. https://doi.org/10.1016/j.infbeh.2017.03.003.

25. Nyqvist KH, Rosenblad A, Volgstern H, Funkquist E-L, Mattsson E. Early skin-to-skin contact between healthy late preterm infants and their parents: an observational cohort study. Peer J. 2017;5:e3949. https://doi.org/10.7717/peerj.3949.

26. Belsky J, Pluess M. Beyond diathesis stress: differential susceptibility to environmental influences. Psychol Bull. 2009;135(6):885–908. https://doi.org/10.1037/a0017376.

27. Monroe SM, Simons AD. Diathesis-stress theories in the context of life-stress research: implications for depressive disorders. Psychol Bull. 1991;110:406–25. https://doi.org/10.1037//0033-2909.110.3.406.

28. Gueron-Sela N, Atzaba-Poria N, Meiri G, Marks K. The caregiving environment and developmental outcomes of preterm infants: diathesis stress or differential susceptibility effects? Child Dev. 2015;86(4):1014–30.

29. Zimmerman FJ, Gilkerson J, Richards JA, Christakis DA, Xu D, Gray S, Yapanel U. Teaching by listening: the importance of adult-child conversation to language development. Pediatrics. 2009;124(1):342–9. https://doi.org/10.1542/peds.2008.2008-2267.

30. Caskey M, Stephens B, Tucker R, Vohr B. Adult talk in the NICU with preterm infants and developmental outcomes. Pediatrics. 2014;133(3):e578–84. https://doi.org/10.1542/peds.2013-0104.

31. Pancsofar N, Vernon-Feagans L, The Family Life Project Investigators. Fathers' early contributions to children's language development in families from low-income rural communities. Early Child Res Q. 2010;25(4):450–63.

32. Charpak N, Ruiz-Peláez JG. Resistance to implementing kangaroo mother care in developing countries, and proposed solutions. Acta Paediatr. 2007;95(5):529–34. https://doi.org/10.1111/j.1651-2227.2006.tb02279.x.

33. Bronfenbrenner U. Ecology of the family as a context for human development: research perspectives. Dev Psychol. 1986;22(6):723–42.

34. Abidin R. Parenting Stress Index: Professional Manual. 3rd ed. Lutz, FL: Psychological Assessment Resources; 1995.

35. Misri S, Reebye P, Milis L, Shah S. The impact of treatment intervention on parenting stress in postpartum depressed mothers: a prospective study. Am J Orthopsychiatry. 2006;76(1):115–9. https://doi.org/10.1037/0002-9432.76.1.115.

36. Leigh B, Milgrom J. Risk factors for antenatal depression, postnatal depression and parenting stress. BMC Psychiatry. 2008;8:24. https://doi.org/10.1186/1471-244X-8-24.

The Social Organization of Nurses' Work with Late Preterm Infants in Non-tertiary Care Settings: Out of the Corners of Nurses' Eyes

5

Catherine Ringham, Janet M. Rankin, Shahirose Sadrudin Premji, and Lenora Marcellus

I[1] began my career in neonatal nursing in the 1980s when the margin of viability hovered around 28 weeks' gestational age and infants born at 32–34 weeks balanced on the precipice of life and death with serious respiratory disease. In the years since, the landscape of neonatal care has changed with advancing technologies and better knowledge of neonatal physiology. We have a clearer understanding of the inherent risks and complications of being born preterm, and care is increasingly focused on preventing short- and long-term health problems. Now infants born in the late preterm period (34–36 6/7 weeks' gestational age) have lower mortality rates notwithstanding persistent preterm-related complications. In light of the shifting terrain of neonatal care and unrelenting risks of late preterm birth, our knowledge of the organization and coordination of late preterm infant (LPI) care needs to be better understood.

The clinical research that informs this chapter arose from my curiosity about the uniqueness of Level 2 neonatal care, the type of NICU where LPIs are primarily admitted. Level 3 NICUs provide acute medical and nursing care for extremely fragile infants, whereas Level 2 units are designed as less intense, transitional care environments where preterm and convalescing infants grow and learn to feed before

---

[1] First author Ringham uses the first person "I" throughout this chapter to reference her personal experiences of NICU. We use "our" and "we" to reference the research and analysis on from which this chapter arises.

C. Ringham (✉) · J. M. Rankin
Faculty of Nursing, University of Calgary, Calgary, AB, Canada
e-mail: clringha@ucalgary.ca; jmrankin@ucalgary.ca

S. S. Premji
School of Nursing, Faculty of Health, York University, Toronto, ON, Canada
e-mail: premjis@yorku.ca

L. Marcellus
School of Nursing, University of Victoria, Victoria, BC, Canada
e-mail: lenoram@uvic.ca

© Springer International Publishing AG, part of Springer Nature 2019
S. S. Premji (ed.), *Late Preterm Infants*, https://doi.org/10.1007/978-3-319-94352-7_5

being discharged home. However as I have seen throughout my career, the kind of care in Level 2 NICUs is not as simple as portrayed by the term transitional care. There are many competing demands that nurses must manage. In a relatively mundane rhythm of infant feeding, medication delivery, parent teaching, and so on, nurses' work is frequently punctuated by moments of crisis when critically ill infants need urgent intervention or the overall acuity of the unit overwhelms current resources. While the character of nurses' work can be episodic, infants need to be fed regularly and with careful attention to their immature neurodevelopment. How does this happen inside of the competing demands that nurses' encounter in their work? The focus of this chapter is to illustrate nurses' care of LPIs, to show how infant feeding is a primary focus of their work in Level 2 NICUs, and to understand how feeding work is organized by opposing institutional practices.

In Calgary, Alberta, preterm infants may be admitted to any one of three Level 2 NICUs, to a Level 3/4 tertiary care center, or to the surgical unit at the Children's Hospital for Southern Alberta. The ethnographic data presented in this chapter centers on observations and interviews with Karen,[2] a nurse in a Level 2 center in the city. Karen brings to light the concerns that I experienced in my practice as a neonatal nurse. She tells her account of caring for LPIs and having to make critical decisions about feeding, medication delivery, and following rules that interfered with her ability to provide safe, evidence-based care for her patients. These are stories that drive me to ask and research how the care of LPIs is coordinated by evidence-based policies and guidelines in Alberta and beyond.

LPIs are in the NICU because of their *risk* of complication, not necessarily because they are sick. They demand a different type of nursing and medical care; close observation, delicate handling, and surveillance, rather than technologically intense care. Feeding is a primary focus for LPIs who are otherwise physiologically stable but at significant risk for feeding issues and poor growth patterns. Research demonstrates that, for preterm infants, oral feeding skills are acquired gradually and with attention to an infant's stage of developmental their distinct feeding cues [1].

As with all areas of healthcare, in the Level 2 NICU setting, the quality and safety movement dominates our attention with evidence-based clinical practice documents that direct nursing care. The underlying format of evidence-based protocols is to focus on selective practices thought to be adaptable to detailed, stepwise, pre-planned directions. We suggest that the nature of nurses' work is characterized by the unexpected, frequent interruptions and the irregular demands of each unique infant/family case and is disrupted by safety work that is dominating healthcare settings. The introduction of safety practices may take priority over the hands on care of infants, as you will see in Karen's stories. We uncover how Karen's work of feeding infants is both prominent and invisible in the daily routine of the Level 2 NICU. We describe Karen's approach to support evidence-based feeding practices and show how her knowledge and skills work to provide the best possible care to her patients. This chapter illustrates how new policy documents intended to improve safe patient care actually work against what nurses are trying to achieve: safe, individualized care.

---

[2] Karen is one of the nurse participants in this research. Karen and the names of the infants described in this chapter are pseudonyms.

5.1 Late Preterm Infants and Level 2 NICU Care

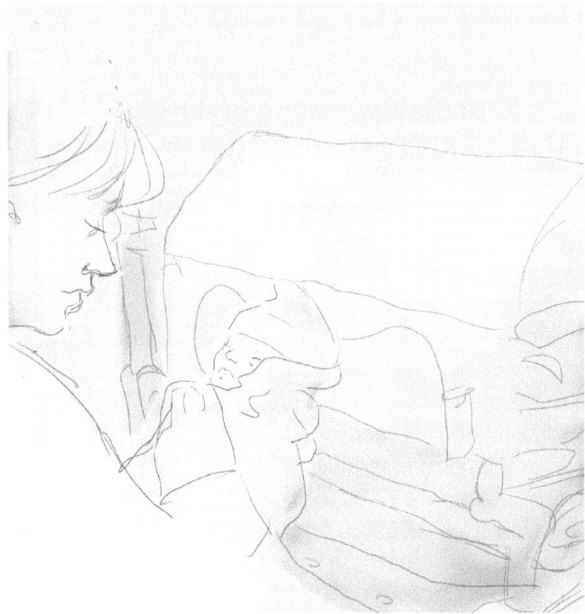

Neonatal care is "levelled" across four classifications of service, Levels 1–4 progressing from low to high acuity. Such categories ensure that resources are appropriately administered and that acutely ill infants and their families have access to centralized specialty resources [2]. A Level 2 nursery provides care for infants generally born late preterm, infants who are recovering from serious medical conditions, and those who were born extremely or very low birth weight who have transitioned out of Level 3 and 4 of NICUs. An infant in a Level 2 NICU is not expected to require ready access to the full range of neonatal or pediatric medical subspecialties, complex respiratory support, or advanced imaging [3, 4]. Level 2 NICUs admit diverse populations of infants, and this creates the unique challenge of mobilizing resources effectively particularly for nursing care [5]. Nurses in Level 2 units provide care for relatively well infants like LPIs while also being called upon to attend the delivery of seriously ill term and preterm infants. As well, Level 2 infants recovering from serious illness can deteriorate and require more intensive care that requires transfer back to a tertiary center. Nurses in Level 2 assist during the stabilization and transfer of these very sick infants.

Where does the LPI fit into NICU health services and within the episodic character of nurses' work? Nursing resources in NICUs are established by global standards, with a set number of nurses scheduled for each shift [6–8]. Ensuring that there are adequate nursing resources in Level 2 NICUs is especially challenging because these nurseries are often small with only a few nurses with the specialty training and experience to provide care to acutely ill infants. In light of the LPIs need for close observation and attention to their risks, nursing resources can be stretched and may compromise safe, individualized patient care.

5.2 What Is Actually Happening in the Care of LPIs? An Ethnographic Account of Nurses' Work

This study traces nurses everyday work activities from frontline care in the Level 2 NICU into institutional policies and practices that coordinate their work in discordant ways. We unexpectedly discovered, through field observations and nurse's accounts of their moment to moment activities, that feeding work was a primary coordinator of activity in the NICU. The need to feed infants was central in almost all nursing work processes. To illustrate how feeding is an essential hub of nurses' work, consider an experienced NICU nurse Karen and her approach to caring for three LPIs during her shift of work.

Karen arrives at the bedside to take report from the night shift nurse; she makes notes on her paper identifying when feeds and medications are due, the volume and method of feedings for each infant, and any anticipated treatments or procedures that she would need to coordinate. She glances toward each of her assigned patients to see if they are awake and alert or still asleep. Karen makes plans to feed Samera first, followed by Sophia, and then Colin. While Karen's planning seems to be straightforward, she recognizes that the babies may wake early for feeding. She also has several medications to administer and knows that the medication procedure "takes a lot of nursing time." In addition, the charge nurse comes by to ask Karen what coffee and lunch breaks she would like. After a quick calculation of the tasks at hand, Karen decides to take the latest break times. She is also reminded by the charge nurse that time-sensitive electronic forms need to be completed and submitted. There are a myriad of other responsibilities that nurses like Karen attend to throughout the course of their day: patient and administrative documentation, reporting at unit rounds, checking equipment, stocking bedsides, and so on. Karen turns her focus toward Samera who is wriggling and sucking on her fist, an indication that she is waking and hungry.

For more than a decade, there has been a proliferation of studies and discussion papers showing the benefits of "cue-based" infant feeding. Across these papers, researchers discuss the significance of attentive observation of infant behavior in order to develop individualized approaches to feeding each unique infant [1, 9–22]. Cue-based feeding practices are built on an infant's neurodevelopmental maturity. There are standard features that underpin good feeding practices for preterm and critically ill infants. Many NICUs now use the evidence that supports infant-led feeding to develop feeding guidelines and protocols to standardize feeding approaches and practice. These are tools for physicians, nurses, and others to assess, direct, and produce ideal feeding experiences [16, 20, 23–25].

Karen knows about infant-led feeding and the implications of either not attending to a preterm infant's cues promptly or pushing oral feeds in instances where the infant is not developmentally ready. She states, "These kids can develop oral aversion and they will shut down and choke because they are not coordinated enough. If you don't pay attention you can really cause problems." For Samera, Karen explains that she is a baby who readily signals to be fed but tires very easily. Taking cues from Samera, Karen suggests, is key to creating a positive experience that will support skill development and competent feeding.

With Karen's knowledgeable and discerning approach, she describes the complex process for introducing a nipple-feeding experience to Samera: "Place the baby on a pillow, on their side and then carefully pace the feed by tipping the nipple to one side or removing it every few sucks. This gives the baby an opportunity to pace themselves and stay organized with their suck/swallow coordination." Samera manages to take a small amount of milk by nipple and then shows Karen signs of disengagement: spilling milk from the corners of her mouth, a disorganized suck, and coughing. An important focus of neonatal nursing care is to support babies to master independent, self-regulated feeding skills [12, 22, 26–29] as Karen described. If Karen had continued with pushing the infant to feed, she would not have supported Samera's state of regulation and might have compromised her future nipple-feeding experiences, so she stopped the feed. The remainder of the milk for infants like Samera is usually given by gavage tube, primarily on a syringe pump over a set period of time. Karen proceeded with setting up this system.

Research shows that positive feeding experiences contribute to appropriate social, emotional, and cognitive development [1, 26, 29]. Nurses like Karen are taught that an infant's feeding skill and competence, the physical coordination of sucking, swallowing, and breathing, and the social interaction involved with feeding are foundational during the neonatal period [17, 22, 30] and also in future growth and development [15, 18, 31–33]. Karen's knowledge of the science of infant feeding, her tacit knowledge, and her skill with flexing her nursing care are evident.

Karen proceeds with completing Samera's feed as Sophia begins to stir in her cot. At the same time, Karen glances at the clock and says she needs to give Colin his medication before Sophia's feed is due. Karen fills a syringe with milk, places it on the feeding pump, and attaches the tubing to Samera's indwelling gavage tube. However, the pump does not infuse when Karen presses the start button. She resets the syringe and tries again. After numerous attempts, Karen powers off the pump and restarts it making it necessary for her to reenter the feeding parameters into the program before pressing start. The milk begins to infuse. Karen comments that she needs to move on to preparing the medication infusion for Colin or "it will be late, and that will be a medication error." Karen is aware that while attending to feeding cues is critical to the infant, the medication policy demands that medications be given within strict parameters or there may be consequences for her and her patient. The organization of infant care in the NICU requires careful planning and relies on the capacity of nurses to mediate institutional processes that coordinate their activities, manage equipment issues, and be attentive to their patients who are unable to overtly articulate their needs.

Later in Karen's day, she describes an instance where she was double-checking a medication with a colleague according to institutional policy. The required safety check occurred while she was in the midst of feeding one of her patients. The medication was being delivered intravenously through a pump that had been preset for the first stage of medication delivery and already double-checked. The pump alarm took precedence when it rang with an alert that required two nurses (according to unit policy) to read the screen again, to reset the program to infuse the next stage of delivery, and to restart the infusion. Karen had to turn her attention to the pump to verify that the medication delivery was correct and reset the pump to infuse again. She described how this played out: "I was the second checker for a med. And I had this baby who was on SINC[3]...a fragile feeder. The baby needed my full attention so I could monitor and read the baby's cues. Well, I was up and down 5 times during that feed. It took me 50 min to complete it...with a fragile baby! They need to be set up properly for the feed like I said before. So, when I had to get up several times during the feed, put the kid in the cot, walk over to the other side of the pod and check the med and syringe pump with the other nurse, it was very disruptive. The baby lost the flow of the feed. Five times!!! *I felt like I was cuing the med, not the baby!*" While Karen's priority is feeding the baby based on how she understands cue-based feeding, the medication delivery policy and the syringe pump alarm make her intention to provide safe feeding care for the infant virtually impossible.

Safety measures, like medication policies that are introduced into the highly technical NICU environment, are often decided *away* from the actual setting—established within abstract plans about what *could* go wrong. What *actually* happens in the NICU drops out of view within institutional constructions of risk, quality, and safety being imposed on nurses. The delicate work of feeding that requires a nurse's full attention, but that is simultaneously considered rather mundane, migrates to the periphery of nurses' attention. The technology seems always to supersede the baby.

5.3   The Social Organization of Feeding in the NICU

5.3.1   Cue-Based Feeding

"Cue-based" or "infant-directed/led" feeding is a practice that has resulted in widely adopted protocols and guidelines across NICU settings [16, 20, 23–25, 34]. This approach to feeding, which we allude to in Karen's account of nursing work, involves "an infant giving cues using physiological signals, as well as motor and state systems (neurobehavioral maturation), to let caregivers know when to offer non-nutritive and nutritive oral feeding experiences" [1]. A cue is an important gesture, a reading of a preterm infant's physical and neurological development that requires experience, knowledge, and time to observe in infant's often subtle signals [1, 12, 30].

---

[3] SINC is a feeding regime, "safe individualized nipple-feeding competence," that offers a stepwise procedure for introducing oral feeding to some preterm infants in the unit where field observations for this study took place.

Researchers from various disciplines have tied together the neurodevelopmental, physiological, and pragmatic aspects of feeding practices and produced evidence that preterm infants demonstrate subtle signals that they are ready to engage in oral stimulation, indicators that are important to developing individualized plans of care [26, 27, 35–38]. Cue-based feeding that is contingent on the observations of astute care providers reportedly optimizes the developmental maturation of preterm and sick infants admitted to NICU [1, 30, 39].

Within the compelling discourse of cue-based infant feeding, nursing work is expected to focus, at least theoretically, on creating a physiologically and neurologically safe, nurturing environment for infants. It is presumed that a plan of care organized in relation to an infant's gestational age at birth will meet the unique developmental needs of each infant [23]. Nurses pay close attention to infants' feeding cues among many other responsibilities including careful monitoring, managing technologies, and documentation. LPIs are at significant risk for feeding issues and therefore require particular surveillance of their feeding behavior. Some LPIs are capable of initiating and sustaining feeding skills and demonstrating feeding competency. Some LPIs take allotted quantities of milk orally and gain weight consistently, while other LPIs do not have the maturity to self-moderate cues or the mechanics of sucking, swallowing, and breathing patterns [10]. Nurses' specialized knowledge of fetal and infant development, and the special needs of LPIs, helps them to predict and respond to each infant's needs in each unique situation [1, 20, 22–24]. Karen's capacity to make consistent observations of Samera's subtle developmental cues illustrates her depth of knowledge and critical decision-making.

Karen's ability to respond within the brief interval of an infant's readiness display is dependent on her having knowledge, experience, and *time*. What we know about Karen's time is that cue-based feeding was derailed by equipment breakdown, the requirement to give medications on time, and the demands of safe feeding practices among many other competing demands. Karen was under pressure to comply with institutional rules that could not accommodate her knowledge about what was actually going on. Despite a carefully crafted care plan, the NICU environment and its many safety rules actually *precluded* Karen and her colleague's capacity to use their judgment during feeding. The numerous protocols that accompany the increasingly technological systems designed to prevent errors do not always intersect effectively with the practices that are intended to provide individualized, safe, and evidence-based infant feeding.

5.3.2   Protocols and Guidelines

Nurses and physicians welcome clinical practice tools such as protocols and guidelines to support decision-making for care NICU patients [1, 40]. These tools aim to standardize care across NICUs and health regions, to ensure there are standard competencies in practices such as feeding approaches, medication delivery, and safe handling of expressed breast milk (EBM) [23, 41, 42]. Standardized clinical practice documents can create tensions for clinicians when they are designed to satisfy the seemingly divergent interests of administrators, physicians, and frontline care providers. The problem is in not seeing and understanding nurses' moment-to-moment actions and decisions in the care of their patients in a NICU environment where work and patient priorities are constantly shifting.

For example, in order to mitigate errors in giving the wrong EBM to the wrong infant, elaborate tracking systems have been instituted in many NICUs. Such systems of accounting for each mother and infant's expressed breast milk follow a dominant logic about safety that imagines that *systems* are the only way to prevent mistakes. In the EBM tracking system, the risk of error is expected to be addressed by electronic barcoding and tracking the whereabouts of a bottle of EBM at any given moment. High-level policies require nurses to adhere closely to the systems intended to ensure safe delivery of EBM. However, these systems cannot possibly accommodate what nurses know is going on in the caregiving moment. These systems overrule nurses' knowledge about critical features of direct patient care. This critical hour-to-hour and day-to-day knowledge and activity is impossible to measure and thus remains *outside* the dominant ideas about what constitutes safe practice. In systems such as these, the institutional rules that dictate that EBM must be managed according to policy eclipses nurses' discretionary knowledge about an individual infant. Flexibility is limited.

In the study being reported in this chapter, the problem of how rules are misaligned with practical knowledge about what is needed in each moment of patient care was particularly apparent on an occasion of a nurse working within the strict protocols of EBM administration. An infant's mother was pumping breastmilk at her baby's bedside for her baby who had been put to the breast for a short time. The mother was now waiting for the nurse to prepare the remainder of the volume of milk to be given via gavage tube. The infant's mother handed the bottle of her freshly pumped milk to the nurse to give to her baby. However, before the EBM could be administered, it had to be registered in the EBM tracking system as "received," a label printed and placed on the bottle, and then the correct amount measured into another bottle. The second bottle then had to be labelled and scanned in the system as "prepare feed." Then the bottle was scanned again to verify the final step as "feed the baby" before the infant could be fed. The EBM tracking system is intended to prevent the chance of error. However, the nurse witnessed the mother pump the milk into a bottle and knew it came from her. The many steps taken to verify the milk within the system took significant time for the nurse and the baby waiting for the milk to be fed. What the nurse knew to be safe and risk-free administration of the EBM in this situation was at odds with the authorized process of tracking and checking written in the safe handling of EBM policy. This policy that underpins precise procedures that determine "safe" practice and aims to prevent errors simply did not make sense in this moment of this competent nurse's practice. It drew her attention to the technology and away from the intimacy that the mother and baby's feeding experience had generated. Those aspects of infant and family care that are immeasurable and critical to well-being are not included in the contemporary organization of safe and efficient NICU care. They are consistently "tacked on" as the individual responsibilities of caring nurses, while at the same time they are being systematically eroded.

Circuits like the EBM tracking system are a type accountability of formal accounting and surveillance that standardizes practices and processes across healthcare to ensure safe care. In the NICU these circuits not only include tracking EBM in nurses' work of feeding but also maintaining technologies associated with medication delivery and following protocols and policies directed at infant feeding practices.

5.4   The Social Organization of Evidence-Based Practice, Quality Improvement, and Safety in NICU: Cue-Based Feeding Subordinated

The organization of neonatal care is underpinned by the logic of order and governance built into technology and clinical practice documents that establish and provide standardized directions for decision-making in practice and across institutions. In the NICU standardizing practices can be seen in each policy, protocol, guideline, and activity that nurses do. Many documents that are produced across levels of healthcare administration regulate how particular aspects of care are provided. Yet these written materials are often disconnected from one another, creating competing rules that impact how nurses can perform safe patient care. Protocols and policies that regulate (and standardize) care assume that each infant, each assessment, and each intervention can be pre-planned, directed, and supported in isolation from the multitude of other things that are going on. However, the nature of nurses' work is characteristically unpredictable and changeable [43, 44]. Over a shift of work in the NICU, there are some activities that have a sense of routine or rhythm: the timing of infant assessments and scheduled feeding, for example. While nurses have some predictability about their work, the inherent nature of the bodily care of infants and the concurrent work with parents have a sense of orderly disorder. Managerial technologies that require nurses to proceed using stepwise structures within matching systems of documentation and record keeping have a logic that attempts to put order into a complex system. The managerial approach of providing "solutions" to problems [45–48] often produces competing demands that care providers mediate with considerable agility.

Despite a great deal of effort directed toward enhancing efficiencies in nursing workflow, evidence-based policies and guidelines remain siloed—each new piece of evidence contributes to the textual "soup" that culminates inside nurses' practice. Thus, the prominent texts (such as clinical practice guidelines and safety policies) that organize feeding are multiple and varied. Despite nurses' efforts to integrate and streamline, the activation of these texts inside the day-to-day unfolding of each unique caregiving circumstance is often disparate and contradictory.

Nurses' feeding work became a focus for the inquiry being reported here when Karen revealed incongruences between the feeding literature, guidelines, protocols, policies, and local feeding practices. Although there were institutional systems developed to ensure that governance documents were integrated, standardized, and streamlined, data from this study revealed how each document was generated independently, during different time frames, and by different people. Karen clearly showed how feeding documents did not coordinate well with one another *or* with the realities of nurses' feeding work. The data arising from the examination of disparate practices and processes demonstrated how nurses' important knowledge was organized and frequently suppressed within the current approaches to the governance of healthcare. Karen illustrated that the proliferation of protocols and guidelines may be *part of the problem*. The context of guideline development siloed and (as this study showed) exacerbated the way that texts competed with important nursing knowledge that nurses like Karen generated from "being there," seeing, touching, and communicating with their patient.

Ultimately, in this study that set out to explore nurses' feeding work with LPIs, serious disconnects were identified between the institutional processes (safe medication administration policies and EBM tracking systems), the ideologies (quality and safety initiatives related to medication and EBM delivery) that dominate the development of textual systems of clinical practice (medication administration records, accurate documentation on the flowsheet, handling EBM and using the system that tracks and audits its administration), and the "care-in-the-moment" approach required by infants from nurses. Our goal was to examine how these complexes of textual coordination—the tracking system for EBM and standardization of documentation for feeding, for example—play out in actions that accomplish safe, competent, *attentive* patient care.

These findings amplify our understanding and appreciation of the episodic and contingent nature of nursing work, perhaps even more so in the Level 2 NICU environment. In addition, the findings draw attention to contested knowledge related to feeding infants in the NICU. That is the critical, practical knowledge nurses have to know what infants need from caregivers, to learn to feed and have the best outcomes possible. What nurses know is frequently incongruent with the plethora of technologies and safety mechanisms constantly introduced into practice, to such a degree that quality and safety are paradoxically compromised. We describe a sense of absurd disorder that emerged as nurses navigated protocols, completed charting, conducted safety checks, and adhered to time-consuming practices that were collectively expected to result in medication safety. Often in this milieu of activity (so it seemed), the infants were viewed "out of the corner of nurses' eyes," socially organized to be rendered peripheral to nurses' full attention. The extensive use of clinical technology and the surveillance required to support this technology establishes its priority in nurses' work. It is an insidious incursion into what nurses might otherwise know and do. It was apparent that, while technologies are intended to increase nurses' capacity to be "safe," nurses like Karen described how technology complicated her work and undermined what she knew about safety. This disjuncture may arise within each priority of care in any moment of practice. Karen showed that her efforts to align feeding science with her observed practice created a disjointed form of feeding work. Although a significant focus of neonatal nurses' everyday work is feeding babies, the actualities of how feeding happens are often invisible.

Conclusion

Feeding, as a nucleus of patient care in the NICU, happens against a backdrop of often highly technical medical intervention and a myriad of institutional technologies, rules, and regulations. Within this technological milieu, LPIs must learn to feed, and parents must learn how to support their fragile infants to feed, grow, and develop neurologically. NICU nurses are key facilitators in the feeding work that is central to neonatal care [1]. Yet, despite (or because of) the policies, guidelines, and doctors' orders that have proliferated with feeding science, nurses' actual work and knowledge of feeding is systematically downgraded in the NICU setting. The time-consuming processes that rapidly expanding technologies have introduced into neonatal care encroach into the time that nurses have to attend to sick and preterm infants. This finding seems particularly relevant for the LPIs who were the original focus of this institutional ethnography. The textual and clinical technologies that pull nurses' attention away from feeding (EBM tracking, medication libraries, syringe pumps that deliver medications, electronically monitored glucometers, and so on) are powerful organizers. They substantially reduce the time and attention nurses can give to the actual infants, especially to those patients whose condition appears stable and whose needs cannot be built into protocols and algorithms, who do not "alarm," and whose actual care does not fit the logics of the proliferation of quality improvement science and safety systems. One of the key findings of this study is that safely feeding fragile infants takes attentive 1:1 time. Although this finding appears self-evident, it is emphasized here to accentuate how nurses' time and attention are being absorbed by institutional accountability systems that pull nurses away from infants and their families.

NICU nurses' attention is frequently diverted from the individual needs of babies. A compelling piece of data that was used to build this argument is Karen's account of the occasion when she is absorbed in the work of feeding a preterm baby. Her attention is urgently drawn to the sound of an alarm that alerts her to check the medication pump at another bedside. Karen knows that the medication pump is not her immediate priority; the medication infusion is finished and the flush needs to be set; there is no risk to the infant. Nonetheless, the call of the alarm trumps the baby's immediate feeding needs. The alarm will not stop until Karen silences it. Karen solves the non-urgent issue with the pump, resetting the infusion in accordance with the medication administration procedure. Meantime, the baby's cry that indicates hunger goes unheeded. Moreover, due to the infant's physiological and neurological immaturity, the baby exhausts her fragile reserves, and her cries cease before the machine alarm has been silenced. This vignette highlights how nurses' actions are directed toward practices and procedures that are hooked into clinical and managerial technologies that are organized within policies, procedures, guidelines, and protocols. These are imperatives that seemingly make sense in an environment saturated with quality improvement projects and safe, evidence-based practice guidelines without intending to actually negatively impact the safe, quality care of LPIs.

References

1. Sables-Baus S, DeSanto K, Henderson S, Kunz J, Morris A, Shields L, et al. Infant-directed oral feeding for premature and critically ill hospitalized infants: guideline for practice. Chicago, IL: National Association of Neonatal Nurses; 2013.
2. Stark AR. American Academy of Pediatrics Committee on fetus and newborn levels of neonatal care pediatrics. 2004;114(5):1341–7.
3. Barfield WD, Papile L, Baley JE, Benitz W, Cummings J, Carlo WA, et al. Levels of neonatal care. Pediatrics. 2012;130(3):587–97.
4. Lasswell SM, Barfield WD, Rochat RW, Blackmon L. Perinatal regionalization for very low-birth-weight and very preterm infants: a meta-analysis. JAMA. 2010;304(9):992–000.
5. Ohnstad MO, Solberg MT. Patient acuity and nurse staffing challenges in Norwegian neonatal intensive care units. J Nurs Manag. 2017;25(7):569–76.
6. Sherenian M, Profit J, Schmidt B, Suh S, Xiao R, Zupancic J, et al. Nurse-to-patient ratios and neonatal outcomes: a brief systematic review. Neonatology. 2013;104(3):179.
7. Pillay T, Nightingale P, Owen S, Kirby D, Spencer A. Neonatal nurse staffing and delivery of clinical care in the SSBC Newborn Network. Arch Dis Child Fetal Neonatal Ed. 2012;97(3):F174–F8.
8. Mullinax C, Lawley M. Assigning patients to nurses in neonatal intensive care. J Oper Res Soc. 2002;53(1):25–35.
9. Alderdice F, Craig S, Doran J, Jenkins J, McCall E, McGowan JE. Regional follow up of late preterm neonatal intensive care graduates. Nurse Res. 2012;19:37.
10. Munson M, Saatkamp R, West C. Late preterm infants: steps to success. Neonatal Netw. 2011;30(4):267–70.
11. Briere C, Lucas R, McGrath JM, Lussier M, Brownell E. Establishing breastfeeding with the late preterm infant in the NICU. J Obstet Gynecol Neonatal Nurs. 2015;44(1):102–13.
12. Swant L, Fairchild R. Placing the bottle or breast in their premature hands: a review of cue-based feeding research. J Neonatal Nurs. 2014;20(3):122–8.
13. Briere CE, McGrath J, Cong X, Cusson R. State of the science: a contemporary review of feeding readiness in the preterm infant. J Perinat Neonatal Nurs. 2014;28(1):51.
14. Arayici S, Simsek GK, Dizdar EA, Sari F, Canpolat FE, Oguz S, et al. Feeding difficulty in late preterm infants. Arch Dis Child. 2014;99(10):A442(1).
15. White A, Parnell K. The transition from tube to full oral feeding (breast or bottle) – a cue-based developmental approach. J Neonatal Nurs. 2013;19(4):189–97.
16. McClure D. An evidence-based approach to feeding the late preterm infant. South Orange, NJ: Seton Hall University; 2013.
17. Jones LR. Oral feeding readiness in the neonatal intensive care unit. Neonatal Netw. 2012;31(3):148–55.
18. DeMauro SB, Patel PR, Medoff-Cooper B, Posencheg M, Abbasi S. Postdischarge feeding patterns in early- and late-preterm infants. Clin Pediatr. 2011;50(10):957–62.
19. Ludwig SM. Oral feeding and the late preterm infant. Newborn Infant Nurs Rev. 2007;7(2): 72–5.
20. Premji SS, McNeil DA, Scotland J. Regional neonatal oral feeding protocol: changing the ethos of feeding preterm infants. J Perinat Neonatal Nurs. 2004;18(4):371–84.
21. Messer LL. Infant-driven feeding vs. scheduled feeding: the effect on hospital length of stay. Minneapolis, MN: Walden University; 2016.
22. Wellington A, Perlman JM. Infant-driven feeding in premature infants: a quality improvement project. Arch Dis Child Fetal Neonatal Ed. 2015;100:F495–500.
23. Kish MZ. Improving preterm infant outcomes: implementing an evidence-based oral feeding advancement protocol in the neonatal intensive care unit. Adv Neonatal Care. 2014;14(5):346–53.
24. Lasby K, Dressler-Mund D. Making the literature palatable at the bedside: reference poster promotes oral feeding best practice. Adv Neonatal Care. 2011;11(1):17–24.

25. McCain GC, Gartside PS, Greenberg JM, Lott JW. A feeding protocol for healthy preterm infants that shortens time to oral feeding. J Pediatr. 2001;139(3):374–9.
26. Pridham K, Steward D, Thoyre S, Brown R, Brown L. Feeding skill performance in premature infants during the first year. Early Hum Dev. 2007;83(5):293–305.
27. Dodrill P, Donovan T, Cleghorn G, McMahon S, Davies PSW. Attainment of early feeding milestones in preterm neonates. J Perinatol. 2008;28(8):549–55.
28. Shaker CS, Werner Woida AM. An evidence-based approach to nipple feeding in a level III NICU: nurse autonomy, developmental care, and teamwork. Neonatal Netw. 2007;26(2):77–83.
29. Thoyre SM, Shaker CS, Pridham KF. The early feeding skills assessment for preterm infants. Neonatal Netw. 2005;24(3):7.
30. Shaker CS. Cue-based feeding in the NICU: using the infant's communication as a guide. Neonatal Netw. 2013;32(6):404.
31. Kirk AT, Alder SC, King JD. Cue-based oral feeding clinical pathway results in earlier attainment of full oral feeding in premature infants. J Perinatol. 2007;27(9):572–8.
32. Meier P, Patel AL, Wright K, Engstrom JL. Management of breastfeeding during and after the maternity hospitalization for late preterm infants. Clin Perinatol. 2013;40(4):689–705.
33. Hayter MA, Anderson L, Claydon J, Magee LA, Liston RM, Lee SK, et al. Variations in early and intermediate neonatal outcomes for inborn infants admitted to a Canadian NICU and born of hypertensive pregnancies. J Obstet Gynaecol Can. 2005;27(1):25.
34. Viswanathan S, McNelis K, Super D, Einstadter D, Groh-Wargo S, Collin MA. standardized slow enteral feeding protocol and the incidence of necrotizing enterocolitis in extremely low birth weight infants. J Parenter Enter Nutr. 2014;39(6):644–54.
35. Bingham PM, Ashikaga T, Abbasi S. Prospective study of non-nutritive sucking and feeding skills in premature infants. Arch Dis Child Fetal Neonatal Ed. 2010;95(3):F194–200.
36. Crowe L, Chang A, Wallace K. Instruments for assessing readiness to commence suck feeds in preterm infants: effects on time to establish full oral feeding and duration of hospitalisation. Cochrane Database Syst Rev. 2012;4:CD005586.
37. Fucile S, McFarland DH, Gisel EG, Lau C. Oral and nonoral sensorimotor interventions facilitate suck–swallow–respiration functions and their coordination in preterm infants. Early Hum Dev. 2012;88(6):345–50.
38. Mizuno K, Ueda A. The maturation and coordination of sucking, swallowing, and respiration in preterm infants. J Pediatr. 2003;142(1):36–40.
39. Kish MZ. Oral feeding readiness in preterm infants: a concept analysis. Adv Neonatal Care. 2013;13(4):230.
40. Baker B. Evidence-based practice to improve outcomes for late preterm infants. J Obstet Gynecol Neonatal Nurs. 2015;44(1):127–34.
41. Fleischman EK. Innovative application of bar coding technology to breast milk administration. J Perinat Neonatal Nurs. 2013;27(2):145.
42. Vitoux RR, Lehr J, Chang H. Eliminating clinical workarounds through improved smart pump drug library use. Biomed Instrum Technol. 2015;23(Suppl):PMID:26444046.
43. Allen D. Inside 'bed management': ethnographic insights from the vantage point of UK hospital nurses. Sociol Health Illn. 2015;37(3):370–84.
44. Potter P, Wolf L, Boxerman S, Grayson D, Sledge J, Dunagan C, et al. Understanding the cognitive work of nursing in the acute care environment. J Nurs Admin Nurs Admin. 2005;35(7–8):327.
45. Timmermans S, Epstein S. A world of standards but not a standard world: toward a sociology of standards and standardization. Annu Rev Sociol. 2010;36:69–89.
46. Star SL, Lampland M, editors. Reckoning with standards. Ithica, NY: Cornell University Press; 2009.
47. Reay T, Hinings CR. Managing the rivalry of competing institutional logics. Organ Stud. 2009;30(6):629–52.
48. Willis E, Toffoli L, Henderson J, Couzner L, Hamilton P, Verrall C, et al. Rounding, work intensification and new public management. Nurs Inq. 2015;23:158–68.

Am I a Frequent Flyer? Taking Care of Late Preterm Infants and Their Parents in the Community

Mary R. Landsiedel and Shahirose Sadrudin Premji

6.1 Introduction

Late preterm infants (LPIs) experience increased risk of morbidity and mortality in the first year of life and beyond when compared with term infants [1–3]. The risk of morbidity and mortality increases rapidly as gestational age at birth decreases [4]. Risks for the LPI can be intensified by maternal conditions and complications occurring during labor and birth [5]. Ongoing morbidities experienced following discharge from hospital increase health-care utilization such as emergency department visits with LPIs having higher health utilization for specific morbidities (e.g., jaundice, infection, respiratory problems) [6] and higher health-care costs than term infants [6, 7]. Moreover, associated challenges in managing these morbidities and separation as a result of rehospitalization can cause emotional distress (stress, anxiety, depression) for parents, impact maternal confidence in care, and hinder parent-infant interactions [8–11].

Majority of emergency department visits in LPIs are considered to be low-acuity visits with LPIs being discharged home [12]. As such, many of the emergency room visits may be avoidable with effective follow-up care. LPIs, however, when compared to term infants, have higher hospital readmissions in the neonatal and infancy period following discharge from the birth hospital [6]. Research estimates that LPIs are more likely to be readmitted to hospital at a rate of 1.5–3 times more often than term infants [7, 13–17]. The most common reasons for readmission are hyperbilirubinemia (jaundice), feeding challenges, infection or suspected infection, and

M. R. Landsiedel (✉)
Bachelor of Midwifery Program, School of Nursing and Midwifery,
Mount Royal University, Calgary, AB, Canada
e-mail: mlandsiedel@mtroyal.ca

S. S. Premji
School of Nursing, Faculty of Health, York University, Toronto, ON, Canada
e-mail: premjis@yorku.ca

© Springer International Publishing AG, part of Springer Nature 2019
S. S. Premji (ed.), *Late Preterm Infants*, https://doi.org/10.1007/978-3-319-94352-7_6

respiratory distress [6, 16–18]. Factors that increase the risk of readmission for the LPI include being the firstborn child, breastfeeding at the time discharge, male gender for non-breastfed LPIs, history of maternal labor and delivery complications, and being of Asian/Pacific Island descent [13, 15, 16, 19]. LPIs with mothers who have confirmed emotional distress in the postpartum period also experienced increased emergency department visits [20]. Readmission of the LPI may be decreased when initial hospital length of stay is greater than 48 h [21]; however, findings are not consistent [19]. Readmission rates have been reported to be reduced with longer length of stay but only among LPIs delivered by cesarean section [18]. A bilirubin screening test prior to discharge and admission to specialized units for moderately ill and seriously ill infants (i.e., Level II or III nurseries) is also associated with reduced readmission [18]. Of note, LPIs 36 weeks gestation are at increased risk of readmission during the first 2 weeks than LPIs 34 and 35 weeks gestation which was attributed to their delayed discharge after birth [22].

LPI readmission rates vary across hospitals, and these variations continue to exist even after accounting for hospital (e.g., patient volume) and biological characteristics [13]. Diverse approaches in discharge practices and in postpartum follow-up care may contribute to differences in readmission rates across institutions [6, 13]. Reduced risk of readmission has been noted when outpatient community follow-up including lactation support occurs within 24–48 h of discharge [16, 19–21]. The actual follow-up strategies used during follow-up care, however, have not always been explicated [13]. Consequently, in this chapter, we detail our developing knowledge of LPIs that informs strategies for discharge planning and postpartum care in the community.

This chapter will present the magnitude of the most common reasons the LPI is readmitted to hospital, namely, hyperbilirubinemia, infection, and respiratory distress. Pattern(s) of readmission will be detailed where evidence is available. Following a brief account of the underlying morbidity, best practices for discharge planning will be detailed with the goal to identify optimal timing of discharge of the LPI, appropriate teaching for parents, and considerations for follow-up to prevent readmission. The nature of feeding problems of LPIs and challenges in managing these difficulties is beyond the scope of this chapter; the reader is referred to Chaps. 6 and 7. The chapter will conclude with general considerations to ensure maternal well-being and family readiness to care for their LPI at home.

6.2 Why Do I Visit the Hospital Frequently?

Our understanding of outcomes of LPIs following discharge from birth hospital is based on limited literature which suggests that readmission rates among LPIs have increased over time [16, 21]. The first 30 days following discharge from birth hospital appear to be important given the increased rates of readmissions reported among LPIs [16]. A summary of published literature comparing readmission following discharge from the birth hospital identified rates of readmission for jaundice to be higher among LPIs, while readmission rates for non-jaundice causes were similar between LPIs and term infants during neonatal period and infancy [6]. We discuss infection, respiratory distress, as these are the most common non-jaundice-related readmission in LPIs [16].

6.2.1 Hyperbilirubinemia (Jaundice)

Hyperbilirubinemia is reported as the most common reason for readmission of the LPI to hospital in the first week of life [15, 17] complicated by feeding difficulties resulting in dehydration and poor weight gain [16, 17, 22–24]. Readmission for jaundice was increased in LPIs who were not cared for in the NICU, had greater severity of illness, and were male infants [13]. LPIs present with more severe hyperbilirubinemia, and resolution takes longer than in term infants [25, 26]. Risk factors associated with severe hyperbilirubinemia requiring readmission to hospital include breastfeeding without adequate lactation support, discharge prior to 72 h, poor milk intake by the infant, and delay in postpartum follow-up (i.e., at 2 weeks) [25].

Hyperbilirubinemia in LPIs is a result of higher levels of unconjugated bilirubin peaking between day 5 and 7 which is later than in term infants [25–27]. An imbalance between bilirubin production and bilirubin elimination leaves the LPI at greater risk for hyperbilirubinemia [25, 28]. Higher levels of bilirubin are a consequence of ineffective binding of bilirubin to albumin due to decreased levels of albumin leading to delayed uptake and conjugation of bilirubin in the liver [25, 27–29]. LPIs are susceptible to decreased excretion of bilirubin through stool stemming from a lower volume of oral feeds and reduced gastrointestinal motility resulting in less passage of stool [25, 28, 29]. An increase in bilirubin combined with increased permeability of the blood-brain barrier makes the LPI more susceptible to kernicterus and possible brain damage [25, 29].

6.2.1.1 Discharge Planning for Hyperbilirubinemia

Bilirubin levels should be evaluated prior to discharge and plotted on a gestational age risk-specific graph followed by continued assessment in the community [15, 30–32]. The LPIs' bilirubin level should be rescreened by a community care provider within 24–48 h of discharge and repeatedly for the first 10 days [26, 28, 30, 32–34]. It is essential that hyperbilirubinemia be treated promptly in the LPI due to the risk of neurological damage related to increased permeability of the brain attributed to the immaturity of the blood-brain barrier [24–26, 28–31]. Ideally, the health-care provider will have knowledge of risks associated with LPIs including rising and declining patterns of bilirubin levels (i.e., delay in reaching peak bilirubin levels to between day 5 and 7 with some infants peaking beyond these days) [24, 35]. Each contact with a health-care provider should consist of weighing the infant, assessment of effective feeding and hydration, and state of alertness as well as maternal well-being [24, 36]. Frequent lactation support throughout the postpartum period has been demonstrated to decrease complications related to hyperbilirubinemia [24]. It is imperative that feeding frequency (8–10 formula feeds or 10–12 breastfeeds per day) is assessed and reinforced during health-care contact in the postpartum period [36]. Health-care providers should review normal output expectations with parents including changes based on day of life, accurately evaluate infant weight without clothing, and reassess bilirubin levels as required [26, 32, 34, 37]. Signs and symptoms of increasing bilirubin should be reviewed with parents including an increase in sleepiness of the infant, difficulty in waking for feeds, decrease in voids and stools, and increasing yellow color of skin and sclera [24]. Emphasizing the importance of follow-up for LPIs with increasing symptoms and providing direction on when parents should seek medical support will assist in the prevention of severe hyperbilirubinemia and readmission to hospital [36, 37].

6.2.2 Infection

Infection (confirmed or suspected) is the most common reason for readmission in LPIs during the second week of life, while jaundice is the most common reason during the first week [15–18]. Infection can produce symptoms that are subtle and nonspecific including temperature instability, signs of respiratory distress, poor color, increased or decreased heart rate, blood pressure changes, decrease in urine output, irritability, poor feeding, vomiting, high or low blood glucose levels, and an increase in jaundice [26, 38, 39]. These symptoms overlap with other morbidities and are unreliable; however, overlooking symptoms of sepsis can have harmful consequences for the LPI [17, 26, 30, 38, 39]. In clinical nursery setting, investigations for sepsis are completed almost three times more often for LPIs than for a term infant [2, 40]. The number of positive infections, however, has been low implying there is a bias toward investigating LPIs for sepsis [41].

LPIs are at increased risk for infection because of their immature immune systems and incomplete maternal antibody transfer across the placenta decreasing the ability to respond to bacterial and viral attacks resulting in more hospital readmissions [26, 39, 42]. This risk is increased for those infants exposed to maternal bacterial or viral infection in utero or in the process of birth [26, 34]. Maternal infections can lead to preterm pre-labor rupture of membranes or preterm labor leading to infection of the infant prior to or during birth with onset of symptoms within 72 h [26, 34, 43]. LPIs can acquire an infection as a result of exposure in the hospital or following discharge leading to an onset of symptoms greater than 72 h after birth [26, 38, 39, 41]. Late-onset infection (positive culture between 4 and 120 days of life) [41] is often slower in onset and more difficult to treat due to the resistant strains of the organisms responsible for the infection resulting in longer treatment with antibiotics. There is a higher probability of late-onset infection among LPIs born to younger mothers (11–19 years) compared to older mothers (20–29 years) and LPIs with 5-min Apgar scores 0–3 and 4–6 [41]. The authors attributed late-onset infection to intravascular devices based on the most common organism (Gram-positive cocci) causing the infection [41].

6.2.2.1 Discharge Planning for Infection
LPIs can acquire an infection as a result of exposure in the hospital or following discharge leading to an onset of symptoms greater than 72 h after birth [26, 43].

Recognizing the vulnerabilities of the LPI starts in hospital and carries through to the community, health-care providers must educate parents on risks of infection and patterns of morbidities [33]. Providers present at the birth must obtain a detailed history including the presence of maternal fever, prolonged rupture of membranes, suspected maternal infections, as well as fetal heart rate abnormalities and intolerance of labor [26]. Moreover, this information should be communicated to health-care provider in the community to ensure a systematic approach to clinical suspicion for infection to promote targeted identification and management of infection. Assessment of infection in LPIs within the context of the complete clinical picture will limit over investigation of sepsis and readmission. For example, warming a cool baby with skin-to-skin contact and assisting with feeding to ensure effective transfer of milk may eliminate concerning signs of mild respiratory distress, hypothermia, and hypoglycemia preventing readmission.

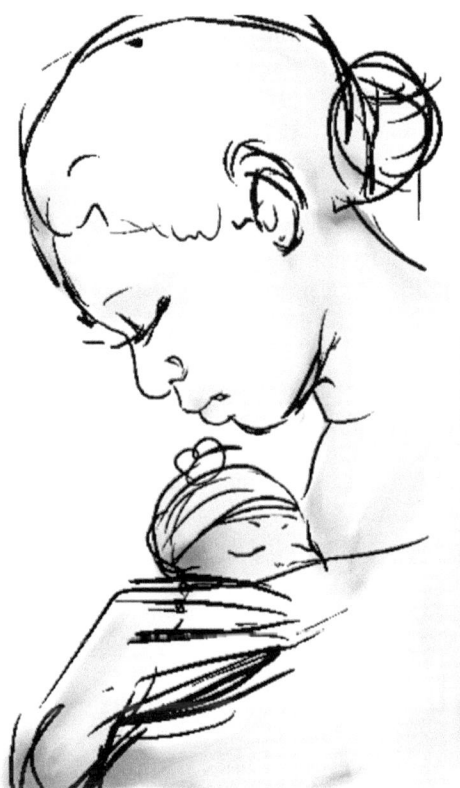

6.2.3   Respiratory Distress

In LPIs, during infancy and early childhood, there is a noticeable increase in readmission for respiratory syncytial virus (RSV) or bronchiolitis when compared to term infants [6]. Respiratory distresses such as bronchiolitis, pneumonia, and RSV were the most common cause for readmission after the first 2 weeks following discharge from birth hospital (i.e., late rehospitalization) [7, 16, 22]. Readmission rates appear to vary between countries [44]. Although RSV leads to rehospitalization among all infants, it appears that the severity of illness is pronounced among LPIs who also require longer hospital stay due to severity of illness and more medical care during their hospitalization than term infants [7, 44–47]. Although clinical manifestations of RSV are similar between premature and term infants—respiratory distress, low-grade fever, cough, and tachypnea—premature infants experience apnea and hypoxemia [44, 47].

Following discharge, LPIs are more susceptible to respiratory distress due to incomplete lung maturation decreasing the infant's oxygen capacity and immaturity of the immune system to fight the infection [45, 46]. LPIs at most risk include those who are born before or during RSV season—usually winter months in North America with varied start, peak, and end periods depending on geographic region— have breastfed for less than 2 months, have preschool or school age siblings, had low birth weight, live in homes where there is smoking, are exposed to crowds or attend daycare, and are male [44, 45]. There are few studies examining RSV multiple risk factors in LPIs—socioeconomic and environmental—which may have additive influence on outcomes of LPIs [44]. Consequently, risk factors may vary from country to country; necessitating tailoring of prevention strategies [48]. Palivizumab prophylaxis though demonstrated to be effective in reducing readmission from RSV bronchiolitis in premature neonates, is not used for all LPIs primarily due to cost [45, 48]. Clinical practice guidelines for palivizumab prophylaxis vary based on epidemiological considerations of RSV [48].

6.2.3.1 Discharge Planning for Respiratory Distress

Parents should receive information about the risk and presenting signs and symptoms of RSV [49, 50]. Parents teaching should highlight prevention strategies including proper hand hygiene for everyone in the home, avoiding contact with people who have symptoms of a cold, benefits of continued breastfeeding, importance of a smoke-free environment, and limiting exposure of the infant to crowds [49, 50]. Health-care providers should be aware of the immunization programs available in their community and refer parents with eligible infants [43, 45, 46, 48, 49].

6.3   General Consideration for Discharge Planning

Discharge planning for the infant from NICU or the postpartum unit begins at admission with close monitoring, support, education and anticipatory guidance surrounding behavior, feeding challenges, and symptoms of illness or concern [51–53]. LPIs discharged early and who have additional risks (e.g., delivered vaginally) will require more intense follow-up, community resources, and continuity of care (i.e., hospital to home to hospital) to ensure safe discharge home (i.e., prevent readmission) [28, 33, 51, 52, 54]. Discharge should be determined based on the LPI's physiological stability (e.g., absence of hyperbilirubinemia), maternal proficiency to identify signs and symptoms of complications requiring medical attention, and maternal psychoso-cial readiness to care for the infant at home [33, 52, 53]. Parents of LPIs who will be discharged directly from the NICU should be offered the opportunity to stay over-night within the hospital and have access to support of nursing staff to assess the family's readiness to care for the infant at home [33]. Consideration must be given to maternal health, ability to effectively breastfeed and/or orally feed the infant, and the availability of support for the dyad at home and in the community [33].

6.4 Maternal Considerations

While assessment of the infant is of prime importance for discharge, maternal well-being and family readiness to care for the infant at home cannot be overlooked. When an LPI has been admitted to NICU following birth, there is an increased risk of postpartum depression especially when there is a longer length of stay coupled with maternal stress, anxiety, and low confidence levels [55]. Mothers of LPIs, when compared to mothers of full-term infants, experience situational anxiety, depression, posttraumatic symptoms, and worry following delivery and at 1 month which is also evident in maternal narratives [56]. The emotional distress is related to the challenges of caring for their LPI [8, 11, 55, 56], especially breastfeeding challenges [8, 11] which are not anticipated given "normalization" of LPIs by care providers [8]. Mothers also report anxiety and stress related to infant behavior [8, 55, 56]. Mothers lack knowledge of feeding issues and other related needs of their LPIs, and inconsistent and contradictory approaches by health-care providers impact maternal confidence in care over time [8]. Lack of readiness to care for LPI, heightened concerns about challenges experienced, decreased confidence, and con-flicting messages from health-care providers may increase health-care utilization [51]. LPIs status combined with diagnosis of maternal mental health doubled the rates of emergency department visits when compared to full-term infants whose mothers have no mental health issue [20]. Screening for mental health issues prior to discharge is imperative to identify LPIs mothers who may be at high risk of emo-tional distress and would benefit from appropriate referral and community supports [55]. We also refer the reader to Chapter 3 which comprehensively examines emo-tional distress during pregnancy and the postpartum period including screening and management. It is essential that information related to both mother and her LPI is documented on the discharge summary and communicated to community health-care providers to facilitate further assessment and continuity of care for the family at home [36, 55, 57]. Fathers play a significant role in the provision of emotional and instrumental support as do family and friends [8]. As such, health-care provid-ers need to be responsive to needs of the father as they are critical to the well-being of the mothers and LPI—see Chap. 4. When it is determined that there is concern for maternal and/or partner mental health, prompt referral to an appropriate profes-sional health-care provider should be initiated to decrease the impact on LPI's development [36, 55, 56] and possibly decrease readmission to hospital for the LPI [20, 51, 55].

Anticipatory guidance particularly with regard to morbidities experienced by LPIs and an integrated multidisciplinary approach to care may promote maternal confidence in care and maternal mental health [11, 53, 57]. Initiating and reinforcing understanding of the unique challenges for LPIs including feeding difficulties, behavioral differences, and developmental delays and guiding parents to use community resources are also important for easier transition to parenthood [8, 36, 53]. Involvement of the family in the care of the LPI and providing education surrounding management of the infants unique challenges leads to empowerment of the family and easier transition from hospital to home [33, 56]. Standardizing approaches to care of LPIs, both in hospital and home, may reduce emotional distress of mothers [8, 52]. Finally, strategies to improve transitions across setting—home to hospital to home—requires innovation in models of care [33] and technology to promote information exchange.

Conclusion

LPIs who are treated as term infants and where clinicians fail to recognize their biological risk are more likely to be readmitted for hyperbilirubinemia and feeding problems increasing the likelihood of neurodevelopmental issues [25]. Although LPIs may meet weight requirements and appear appropriate for care by parent in the postpartum unit, these infants have unique challenges that increase their risk for morbidity, mortality, and readmission to hospital following discharge [1–7]. Delaying discharge of the LPI until appropriate criteria are met including the ability to tolerate oral feeds, increased maternal milk volume is achieved, absence of hyperbilirubinemia as well as assessment of maternal physiological and psychosocial readiness will facilitate successful transition from hospital to home [36, 53, 55, 56]. Continuity of care in the community by health-care practitioners with expertise in care of the LPI is essential for facilitating continuous education and support empowering families to confidently care for their LPI [28, 33, 51, 52, 54, 56]. Regular assessment with primary care practitioners and/or public health nurses will assist in timely recognition of concerns leading to early intervention potentially decreasing the need for readmission to hospital [6, 8]. Evidence-informed guidelines have the potential to reduce emergency department visits and risk of hospital readmission in the first month of life [58].

References

1. Teune MJ, Bakhuizen S, Gyamfi Bannerman C, Opmeer BC, van Kaam AH, van Wassenaer AG, Morris JM, Mol BW. A systematic review of severe morbidity in infants born late preterm. Am J Obstet Gynecol. 2011;205(4):374.e1–9. https://doi.org/10.1016/j.ajog.2011.07.015.
2. Johnston KM, Gooch K, Korol E, Vo P, Eyawo O, Bradt P, Levy A. The economic burden of prematurity in Canada. BMC Pediatr. 2014;14:93. https://doi.org/10.1186/1471-2431-14-93.
3. Mathews TJ, MacDorman MF. Infant mortality statistics from the 2006 period linked birth/infant death data set. Nat Vital Stat Rep. 2010;58(17):1–31.

4. Baslek JA, Sammel MD, Paré E, Srinivas SK, Posencheg MA, Elovitz MA. Adverse neonatal outcomes: examining the risks between preterm, late preterm, and term infants. Am J Obstet Gynecol. 2008;199(4):367.e1–8. https://doi.org/10.1016/j.ajog.2008.08.002.
5. Shapiro-Mendoza CK, Tomashek KM, Kotelchuck M, Barfield W, Nannini A, Weiss J, Declercq E. Effect of late-preterm birth and maternal medical conditions on newborn morbidity risk. Pediatrics. 2008;121(2):e223–32. https://doi.org/10.1542/peds.2006.3629.
6. Isayama T, Lewis-Mikhael AM, O'Reilly D, Beyene J, McDonald SD. Health services use by late preterm and term infants from infancy to adulthood: A meta-analysis. Pediatrics. 2017;140(1):e20170266. https://doi.org/10.1542/peds.207-0266.
7. McLaurin KK, Hall CB, Jackson EA, Owens OV, Mahadevia PJ. Persistence of morbidity and cost differences between late-preterm and term infants during the first year of life. Pediatrics. 2009;123(2):653–9.
8. Premji SS, Currie G, Reilly S, Dosani A, Oliver LM, Lodha AK, Young M. A qualitative study: mothers of late preterm infants relate their experiences of community-based care. PLoS One. 2017;12(3):e.0174419. https://doi.org/10.1371/journal.pone.0174418.
9. Chee CY, Chong YS, Ng TP, Lee DT, Tan LK, Fones CS. The association between maternal depression and frequent non-routine visits to the infant's doctor—a cohort study. J Affect Disord. 2008;107:247–53.
10. Dosani A, Hemraj J, Premji SS, Currie G, Reilly SM, Lodha AK, Young M, Hall M. Breastfeeding the late preterm infant: experiences of mothers and perceptions of public health nurses. Int Breastfeed J. 2017;12:23. https://doi.org/10.1186/s13006-017-01140-0.
11. Tully K, Holditch-Davis D, Silva S, Brandon D. The relationship between infant feeding outcomes and maternal emotional well-being among mothers of late preterm and term infants. Adv Neonatal Care. 2017;17(1):65–75.
12. Jain S, Cheng J. Emergency department visits and rehospitalizations in late preterm infants. Clin Perinatol. 2006;33(4):935–45. https://doi.org/10.1016/j.clp.2006.09.007.
13. Escobar GJ, Greene JD, Hulac P. Rehospitalization after birth hospitalization: patterns among infants of all gestations. Arch Dis Child. 2005;90:125–31. https://doi.org/10.1136/adc.2003.039974.
14. Martens PJ, Derksen S, Gupta S. Predictors of hospital readmission of Manitoba newborns within six weeks postbirth discharge: a population-based study. Pediatrics. 2004;114:708–13. https://doi.org/10.1542/peds.2003-0714-L.
15. Shapiro-Mendoza CK, Tomashek KM, Kotelchuck M. Risk factors for neonatal morbidity and mortality among "healthy", late preterm newborns. Sem Perinatol. 2006;30:54–60. https://doi.org/10.1053/j.semperi.2006.02.002.
16. Kuzniewicz MW, Parker SJ, Schnake-Mahl A, Escobar GJ. Hospital readmissions and emergency department visits in moderate preterm, late preterm and early term infants. Clin Perinatol. 2013;40(4):753–75. https://doi.org/10.1016/j.clp.2013.07.008.
17. Tomashek KM, Shapiro-Mendoza CK, Weiss J, Kotelchuck M, Barfield W, Evans S, Naninni A, Declercq E. Early discharge among late preterm and term newborns and risk of neonatal morbidity. Sem Perinatol. 2006;30(2):61–8. https://doi.org/10.1053/j.sempei.2006.02.003.
18. Moyer LB, Goyal NK, Meinzen-Derr J, Rust CL, Wexelblatt SL, Greenberg M. Factors associated with readmission in late-preterm infants: a matched case control study. Hosp Pediatr. 2014;4(5):298–304. https://doi.org/10.1542/hpeds.2013-0120.
19. Goyal N, Zubizarreta JR, Small DS, Lorch SA. Length of stay and readmission among late preterm infants: an instrumental variable approach. Hosp Pediatr. 2013;3(1):7–15.
20. Goyal NK, Folger AT, Hall ES, Ammerman RT, Van Ginkel JB, Pickler RS. Effects of home visiting and maternal mental health on use of the emergency department among late preterm infants. J Obstet Gynecol Neonatal Nurs. 2015;44(1):135–44.
21. Harron K, Gilbert R, Cromwell D, Oddies S, van derMeulen J. Newborn length of stay and risk of readmission. Pediatr Perinat Epidemiol. 2017;31(3):221–32. https://doi.org/10.1111/ppe.12359.
22. Escobar GJ, Clark RH, Greene JD. Short-term outcomes of infants born at 35 and 36 weeks gestation: we need to ask more questions. Semin Perinatol. 2006;30(1):28–33. https://doi.org/10.1053/j.semperi.2006.01.005.

23. Meier PP, Furman LM, Degenhardt M. Increased lactation risk for late preterm infants and mothers: evidence and management strategies to protect breastfeeding. J Midwifery Womens Health. 2007;52(6):579–87.
24. Smith JR, Donze A, Schuller L. An evidence-based review of hyperbilirubinemia in the late preterm infant, with implications for practice: management, follow-up, and breastfeeding support. Neonatal Netw. 2007;26(6):395–405.
25. Bhutani VK, Johnson L. Kernicterus in late preterm infants cared for as term healthy infants. Semin Perinatol. 2006;30(2):89–97.
26. Darcy AE. Complications of the late preterm infant. J Perinat Nurs. 2008;23(1):78–86.
27. Kaplan M, Muraca M, Vreman HJ, Hammerman C, Vilei MT, Rubaltelli FF, Stevenson DK. Neonatal bilirubin production-conjugation imbalance: effect of glucose-6-phosphate dehydrogenase deficiency and borderline prematurity. Arch Dis Child. 2005;90:F123–7.
28. Mally PV. Clinical issues in the management of late preterm infants. Curr Probl Pediatr Adolesc Health Care. 2010;40(9):218–33. https://doi.org/10.1016/j.cppeds.2010.07.005.
29. Wallenstein MB, Bhutani VK. Jaundice and kernicterus in the moderately preterm infant. Clin Perinatol. 2013;40(4):679–88. https://doi.org/10.1016/j.clp.2013.07.007.
30. Stuckey-Schrock K, Schrock SD. Head off complications in late preterm infants. J Fam Pract. 2013;62(4):E3–8.
31. Kaur S, Chawla D, Pathak U, Jain S. Predischarge non-invasive risk assessment for prediction of significant hyperbilirubinemia in term and late preterm neonates. J Perinatol. 2012;32(9):716–21. https://doi.org/10.1038/jp.2011.170.
32. Barrington KJ, Sankaran K. Guidelines for the detection, management and prevention of hyperbilirubinemia in term and late preterm newborn infants. Pediatr Child Health. 2007;12(Suppl B):1B–12B.
33. Whyte RK. Safe discharge of the late preterm infant. Pediatr Child Health. 2010;15(10):655–60.
34. Souto A, Pudel M, Hallas D. Evidence-based care management of the late preterm infant. J Pediatr Health. 2011;25(1):44–9. https://doi.org/10.1016/j.pedhc.2010.04.002.
35. Engle WA, Tomashek KM, Wallman C. "Late-preterm" infants: a population at risk. Pediatrics. 2007;120(6):1390–401.
36. Phillips RM, Goldstein M, Hougland K, Nandyal R, Pizzica A, Santa-Donato A, Staebler S, Stark AR, Treiger TM, Yost E, On Behalf of The National Perinatal Association. Multidisciplinary guidelines for the care of late preterm infants. J Perinatol. 2013;33(Suppl 2):S5–S22. https://doi.org/10.1038/jp.2013.53.
37. Barkemeyer BM. Discharge planning. Pediatr Clin N Am. 2015;62(2):545–56. https://doi.org/10.1016/j.pcl.2014.11.013.
38. van Herk W, Stocker M, van Rossum AMC. Recognizing early onset neonatal sepsis: an essential step in appropriate antimicrobial use. J Infect. 2016;72(Suppl 5):S77–82. https://doi.org/10.1016/j.jinf.2016.04.026.
39. Cortese F, Scicchitano P, Gesualdo M, Filaninno A, De Giorgi E, Schettini F, Laforgia N, Ciccone MM. Early and late infections in newborns: where do we stand? A review. Pediatr Neonatol. 2016;57(4):265–73. https://doi.org/10.1016/j.pedneo.2015.09.007.
40. Wang ML, Dorer DJ, Fleming MP, Catlin EA. Clinical outcomes of near-term infants. Pediatrics. 2004;114(2):372–6.
41. Cohen-Wolkowiez M, Moran C, Benjamin DK, Cotton CM, Clark RH, Benjamin DK Jr, Smith PB. Early and late onset sepsis in late preterm infants. Pediatr Infect Dis J. 2009;28(12):1052–6.
42. Lott JW. State of the science: neonatal bacterial infection in the early 21st century. J Perinat Neoant Nurs. 2006;20(1):62–70.
43. Hubbard E, Stellwagen L, Wolf A. The late preterm infant: a little baby with big needs. Contemp Pediatr. 2007;24(11):51–8.
44. Carbonell-Estrany X, Figueras-Aloy J, Law BJ, Infección Respiratoria Infantil por Virus Respiratorio Sincitial Study Group Pediatric Investigators Collaborative Network of Infections in Canada Study Group. Identifying risk factors for severe respiratory syncytial virus among infants born after 33 through 35 completed weeks of gestation: different methodologies yield consistent findings. Pediatr Infect Dis J. 2004;23(11 Suppl):S193–201.

45. Resch B, Paes B. Are late preterm infants as susceptible to RSV as full term infants? Early Hum Dev. 2011;87.(Suppl:S47–9. https://doi.org/10.1016/j.earlhumdev.2011.01.010.
46. Helfrich AM, Nyland CM, Eberly MD, Eide MB, Stagliano DR. Healthy late-preterm infants born between 33–36+6 weeks gestational age have higher risk for respiratory syncytial virus hospitalization. Early Hum Dev. 2015;91(9):541–6. https://doi.org/10.1016/j.earlhumdev.2015.06.009.
47. Meert K, Heidemann S, Abella B, Sarnaik A. Does prematurity alter the course of respiratory syncytial virus infection? Crit Care Med. 1990;18(12):1357–9.
48. Lanari M, Silvestri M, Rossi GA. Palivizumab prophylaxis in 'late preterm' newborns. J Matern Fetal Neonatal Med. 2010;23(Suppl 3):53–5. https://doi.org/10.3109/14767058.2010.506757.
49. Robinson JL, Le Saux N. Preventing hospitalizations for respiratory syncytial virus infection. Pediatr Child Health. 2015;20(6):321–6.
50. Jefferson T, Del Mar CB, Dooley L, Ferroni E, Al-Ansay LA, Bawazeer GA, van Driel ML, Nair S, Jones MA, Thorning S, Conly JM. Physical interventions to interrupt or reduce the spread of respiratory viruses. Cochrane Database Syst Rev. 2011;7:CD006207. https://doi.org/10.1002/14651858.CD006207.pub4.
51. Premji SS, Young M, Rogers C, Reilly S. Transitions in the early-life of late preterm infants: vulnerabilities and implications for postpartum care. J Perinat Neonat Nurs. 2012;26(1):57–68. https://doi.org/10.1097/JPN.0b013e21823f8ff5.
52. Quinn JM, Sparks M, Gephart SM. Discharge criteria for the late preterm infant: a review of the literature. Adv Neonatal Care. 2017;17(5):362–71. https://doi.org/10.1097/ANC.0000000000000406.
53. Jeffries AL. Going home: facilitating discharge of the preterm infant. Pediatr Child Health. 2014;19(1):31–6.
54. Hwang SS, Barfield WD, Smith RA, Morrow B, Shapiro-Mendoza CK, Prince CB, Smith VC, McCormick MC. Discharge timing, outpatient follow-up, and home care of late preterm and early term infants. Pediatrics. 2013;132(1):101–8. https://doi.org/10.1542/peds.2012-3892.
55. Hawes K, McGowan E, O'Donnell M, Tucker R, Vohr B. Social emotional factors increase the risk of postpartum depression in mothers of preterm infants. J Pediatr. 2016;179:61–7. https://doi.org/10.1016/j.jpeds.2016.07.008.
56. Brandon DH, Tully KP, Silva SG, Malcolm WF, Murtha AP, Turner BS, Holditch-Davis D. Emotional responses of mothers of late-preterm and term infants. J Obstet Gynecol Neonatal Nurs. 2011;40(6):719–31. https://doi.org/10.1111/j.1552-6909.2011.01290.x.
57. Gallini F, Arena R, Romano V, Frezza S, Romagnoli C. Follow-up of late preterm infants: why, what and who? Ital J Pediatr. 2014;40(Suppl 2):A26. https://doi.org/10.1186/1824-7288-40-S2-A26.
58. Shahid R, Schneck KE, Zimmerman C. Ed visits and hospital readmission of late preterm infants decrease after implementation of practice guidelines. Pediatrics. 2018;141(1):MeetingAbstract. https://doi.org/10.1542/peds.141.1_MeetingAbstract.516.

Breastfeeding the Late Preterm Infant: Supporting Parents with the Challenges of Breastfeeding a Late Preterm Infant

Genevieve Currie, Allison C. Munn, and Sarah N. Taylor

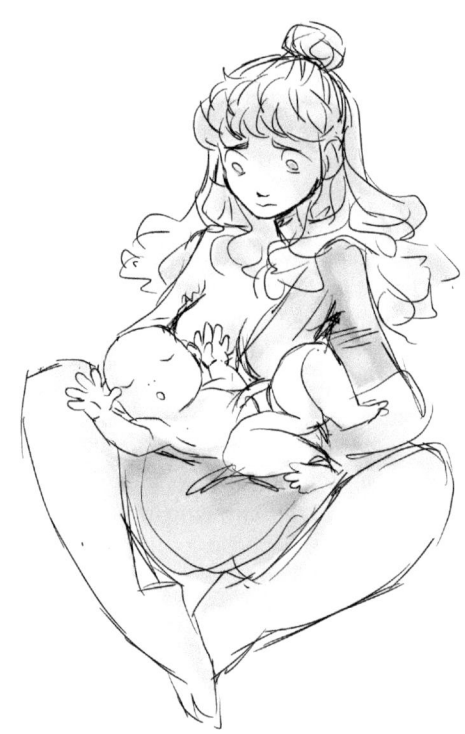

G. Currie (✉)
School of Nursing and Midwifery, Mount Royal University, Calgary, AB, Canada
e-mail: Gcurrie@mtroyal.ca

A. C. Munn
Department of Nursing, Francis Marion University, Florence, SC, USA
e-mail: Amunn@fmarion.edu

S. N. Taylor
Department of Pediatrics, Medical University of South Carolina, Charleston, SC, USA
e-mail: Taylorse@musc.edu

© Springer International Publishing AG, part of Springer Nature 2019
S. S. Premji (ed.), *Late Preterm Infants*, https://doi.org/10.1007/978-3-319-94352-7_7

7.1   Clinical Case Study: Sara's Story

Sara is a 24-year-old primigravida who recently gave birth to a boy she named Samuel. Sara attended prenatal visits regularly and had an unremarkable pregnancy until she began experiencing symptoms of preterm labor at 30 weeks of pregnancy. Sara was admitted to the hospital, where the progression of labor was delayed until 35 weeks of pregnancy, and baby Samuel was delivered via vaginal birth, weighing 6.6 pounds (3000 g). Despite his early arrival, Samuel appeared healthy at birth. He registered Apgar scores of 9 and 9, and he did not exhibit temperature instability or respiratory distress. Sara participated in immediate skin-to-skin contact with Samuel, and breast-feeding was initiated approximately 45 min after delivery. During the postpartum hospital stay, Sara voiced concerns about Samuel falling asleep during breastfeeding sessions. The health care provider (HCP) offered strategies for infant positioning, recognizing hunger cues, promoting a successful latch, and observing for signs of good sucks and swallows. Sara and Samuel were discharged from the hospital within 36 h after delivery. However, by 7 days post-delivery, Sara noticed that Samuel was sleeping excessively and having few wet and dirty diapers and was too weak to latch. Sara took Samuel to the emergency room, where he presented dehydrated with a weight loss of over 10% of his birth weight, and he had an elevated serum bilirubin level. Samuel was admitted to the children's hospital where he received intravenous fluids, phototherapy, and supplemental feedings until he began to gain weight, was more alert, and his bilirubin level decreased. A HCP once again visited Sara and Samuel and discovered that multiple factors contributed to Samuel's readmission, including infant drowsiness, disorganized feeding patterns, a weak ineffective suck, and delayed maternal milk production. The HCP provided specific feeding strategies, tailored to the late preterm infant's needs, to ensure the health and breastfeeding success of Sara and Samuel upon discharge home. Sara and Samuel's story is familiar to practitioners caring for late preterm infants (LPIs). Although, LPIs may appear to be like healthy term infants, they have specific physiological vulnerabilities and increased risk for breastfeeding difficulties and hospital readmission. This chapter will include guidelines to identify breastfeeding difficulties and support mothers and fathers of LPIs in their efforts to successfully and safely feed in the postpartum hospital environment, home, and community.

7.2   Background and Overview of Breastfeeding and Late Preterm Infants

The benefits of breastfeeding are well-documented, with exclusive breastfeeding for 6 months associated with decreased risk for multiple adverse health outcomes, including otitis media, respiratory infections, gastrointestinal conditions, asthma, childhood obesity, sudden infant death syndrome, and maternal breast and ovarian cancers [1, 2]. Preterm infants particularly benefit from the protective features of human milk through decreased risk for sepsis and a potentially fatal gastrointestinal condition, necrotizing enterocolitis [1, 2]. Additionally, human milk improves outcomes for preterm infants through enhanced neurodevelopment and decreased rates of metabolic syndrome in adolescence [1, 2]. LPIs also benefit from exclusive human milk feedings; however, their mothers often struggle to establish and maintain breastfeeding due to physiologic and developmental differences that render LPIs vulnerable to unsuccessful breastfeeding and poor health outcomes [3–7].

LPIs are often known as the "little imposters" [8] because they resemble their full-term counterparts, but they are often physiologically, metabolically, and neurologically immature [9, 10], presenting problems with temperature instability, hypoglycemia, respiratory distress, excessive and extended jaundice, and feeding problems [11]. When these immaturities are not adequately addressed in the early-newborn hospitalization period, LPIs are at an increased risk of morbidity and mortality and rehospitalization within the first 2 weeks after discharge, with complications often relating to feeding difficulties [3, 11]. Specific feeding immaturities include weak, ineffective, and uncoordinated suck and swallow patterns, lack of energy leading to early fatigue with feedings, increased sleepiness, ineffective latch, and inadequate milk transfer [3, 11]. This risk is especially pertinent for breastfed LPIs whose mothers often experience delays in their milk "coming in" and have difficulty establishing and maintaining milk supply [7, 12]. These mothers require additional breastfeeding assessments and support services in the hospital, home, or community environments to promote infant health and successful breastfeeding [3, 11, 13, 14]. Protective interventions include care considerations in the immediate hours after delivery, postpartum hospitalization period [normal newborn care or neonatal intensive care], and experiences in the days, weeks, and months following discharge from the hospital.

7.3 After Birth Experiences: Considerations for Care and Breastfeeding

The Baby-Friendly Hospital Initiative (BFHI) is a World Health Organization (WHO) and UNICEF supported set of evidence-based guidelines to promote breastfeeding in the hospital environment [15]. Interventions associated with the BFHI include the promotion of early skin-to-skin contact, maternal/infant bonding practices, and exclusive breastfeeding [3, 4, 11, 16, 17]. In the clinical case study, baby Samuel did not experience notable physiologic immaturities and complications immediately after birth (e.g., any signs of temperature instability, hypoglycemia, or respiratory distress). Thus, Sara and Samuel had the opportunity to participate in immediate skin-to-skin contact with breastfeeding initiation within the first hour after delivery. This is an appropriate course of care for medically stable LPIs to assist in infant adjustment to extrautcrine life and the facilitation of infant physiologic regulation, infant readiness to initiation breastfeeding, maternal breast stimulation, and maternal/infant bonding [18, 19].

Immediate skin-to-skin contact involves placing the naked infant in a prone position on the mother's bare chest and covering the infant across the back with a warm blanket [19]. Immediate skin-to-skin contact is calming for both the mother and infant, protecting the infant from the negative effects of separation, which aids the infant's ability to self-regulate over time [19]. Additionally, skin-to-skin contact produces maternal release of the hormone oxytocin, promoting bonding and increased maternal self-efficacy and confidence in caring for her child. When a newborn is placed skin-to-skin with the mother for the first hour after birth, the baby progresses through an observable set of behaviors that indicate infant readiness to initiate breastfeeding. Nine behaviors, including "(1) the birth cry, (2) relaxation, (3) awakening, (4) activity, (5) resting, (6) crawling, (7) familiarization, (8) suckling, and (9) sleeping" ([19], p. 70), describe infant adaptation to extrauterine life, familiarization with the mother, instinctive search for the breast, followed by suckling, and ending with a period of sleeping [19, 20].

Skin-to-skin, contact, however, may not be appropriate care for all LPIs because of immaturity and medical instability concerns that place the group at a 50% increased risk for morbidity during the postpartum hospitalization period and often require maternal/infant separation, administration of intravenous fluids, enteral or bottle feedings, and phototherapy [3, 11, 12, 21]. This is particularly significant with breastfeeding because separation may lead to difficulty establishing and sustaining an adequate milk supply from lack of stimulation and thorough milk removal [12, 22]. In addition, LPIs have lower rates of breastfeeding initiation due to limited amounts of skin-to-skin contact within 1 h of delivery, separation due to cesarean section delivery, or maternal medical issues leading to separation after birth [23]. As such, if separation is necessary immediately after birth, Baby-Friendly practice implementation includes early initiation of milk expression in mothers of LPIs. The mother should begin hand expression of colostrum within the first 2 h after delivery to improve maternal milk production and supply [21, 24]. Mothers can express more colostrum with hand expression in the first 48 h than from using an electric breast pump; electric pumps can be used after the first 24 h [25]. Mothers may require several hands-on sessions from HCPs to feel comfortable with hand expression and use of the breast pump. Recognition of delay in effective suckling and milk transfer, necessitating the utilization of breastfeeding supplementation strategies and devices, along with tailored maternal education and breastfeeding support are key to the health and breastfeeding success of LPIs and their parents [3, 12, 22].

7.4 Initiating and Recognizing Effective Suckling and Milk Transfer

Baby Samuel displayed some early warning signs of LPI fatigue and milk transfer insufficiency in the first days after birth. Focused feeding assessments using specific indicators for LPIs could have enhanced Sara's understanding of best breastfeeding practices for Samuel and prevented rehospitalization. Skin-to-skin contact should be initiated as soon as both the mother and infant's conditions are stabilized [21, 26, 27]. Parents can be shown to place their infant skin-to-skin 20–30 min before feedings to rouse and stimulate the infant and initiate early feeding cues [28]. Regular breastfeeds should be encouraged, and it may be necessary to wake the LPI within 2–3 h of the previous feeding to prevent further sleepiness and fatigue, excessive weight loss, and dehydration. LPIs should optimally have 10–12 human milk feedings per 24-h period while closely observing the infant during the first 12–24 h of life for physiologic instability and complications [21]. Providers should assist parents to assess LPIs for cues indicating readiness to feed including hunger cues and successful feeding while on the breast.

Indicators of readiness to feed [29–31]:

- Flexed postural tone.
- Ability to maintain a midline position, with arms and hands held in a forward posture.
- Neurological organizational skills to search for the nipple when it is presented for feeding.
- Ability to coordinate sucking, breathing, and swallowing.

Hunger cues [10, 32]:

- Smacking of the lips.
- Turning the head toward the nipple.
- Hands in the mouth.
- Rooting.
- Clenched fists and rigid arms at the side of the body.

Indicators of successful feeding while on the breast [10, 30, 31]:

- Respiratory effort that is strong, consistent, and within the parameters of normal respirations (30–60 breaths/min). The respiratory rate may be higher at the end of the feeding.
- No labored respirations or skin/mucous membrane color changes.

A LPI should typically spend up to 30 min per feeding session with direct feeding from both breasts or mixed feedings [3]. The parents should be informed that the focus of the feeds is to create a quiet stress-free feeding environment and not focus on volume-driven feeds. Volume-driven feeds can lead to possible regurgitation of feeds, choking, and adverse feeding experiences [33–35].

7.5 Recognizing Feeding Difficulties and Indicators of Unsuccessful Feeding

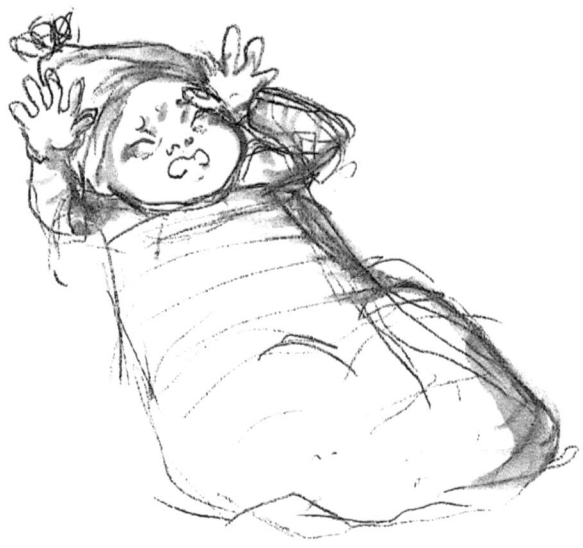

Signs of disorganized feeding [10]:

• Splayed hands and extension of arms away from the body
• Turning away from the nipple or bottle
• Pooling of milk from the mouth
• Skin or mucous membrane color change during a feed
• Arching of the back

At home, Samuel was falling asleep during breastfeeding sessions, sleeping excessively, exhibiting minimal output with few wet and dirty diapers, and was too weak to latch. Feeding assessments and maternal education emphasize that most LPIs lack the physical stamina or maturity to maintain an effective latch and the suck, swallow, and breathe coordination to feed exclusively at the breast [8, 10, 30, 36]. An ineffective suck may appear as subtle oropharyngeal changes with the LPI slightly pulling off the breast sucking on the nipple and audible smacking sounds that indicate an insufficient latch [31]. LPIs indicate their need for respite (i.e., a break) or decrease in stimulation through disengagement cues like turning away from the breast or nipple, arching the back, and falling asleep [32, 35, 37]. Lack of attention to signs of disorganized feeding and difficulties with coordination of suck, swallow, and breath patterns could lead to choking and regurgitation [10].

Expression of colostrum followed by feeding the infant with a spoon, dropper, or other assistive device could ensure adequate intake while preserving infant energy expenditures [3, 21, 27]. Early sensorimotor stimulation to perioral structures such as the cheeks, lips, gums, tongue, jaw, and head, as well as stimulation to the trunk and extremities, can facilitate oral feeding skills and swallowing and breathing coordination [38]. Parents can further support the LPI by:

• Providing side-lying feeding [34].
• Swaddling the LPI with hands out so the infant maintains postural stability and paced feeds [34].
• Using the cross cradle, football or prone positions so the breast can be adequately supported and the infant's mouth and latch can be assessed more easily to determine a deeper latch [8].
• Allowing the LPI to pause between sucks regaining strength to feed and coordinate the suck swallow breath pattern [10].

Feeding assessments should occur at least two times per day by two different HCPs [3, 39]. There are no evidence-informed breastfeeding assessment tools for LPIs, but the LATCH score may provide some prediction of milk intake [40]. The LATCH scoring system includes an evaluation of infant latch, audible swallowing, type of nipple, comfort with breast or nipple, and hold or positioning. LPIs who lose more than 2–3% of birth weight per day or 7% of bodyweight within the first 48–72 h are at risk for dehydration [3, 41]. These infants may not be receiving adequate milk transfer with breastfeeding and consequently have more calorie expenditure relative to milk intake lacking the nutrition required for adequate growth and development [3, 8, 10, 42, 43]. Monitoring and counting wet and dirty diapers can aid in determining adequate milk input: 2 wet and dirty diapers by day 2, 3 wet and dirty diapers by day 3, 4 wet and dirty diapers by day 4, and 6 wet and 4 dirty diapers from day 6 and beyond [3, 44].

Signs of dehydration from inadequate milk transfer [36, 42]:

- Sunken anterior fontanel
- Uric acid crystals after 72 hours of life
- Lethargy
- Decreased urine and stool output

Advising parents to keep a written journal of feedings and wet/dirty diapers helps to ensure an accurate record of the infant's intake and output. The discharge feeding plan should include descriptions and indications for various types of feedings (human milk or infant formula) and method of feeding delivery (breast, cup, bottle, etc.), including supplementation strategies and therapeutic feeding devices (ex. ultrathin silicone nipple shield for direct feeding or feeding tubes and syringes for supplementation). The discharge plan should be based on the feeding plan developed in the hospital and should reflect maternal/family preferences and comfort [3].

7.6   Supplementing with Breast feeding

Sara and Samuel went home within 36 h after delivery. Sara took Samuel to the emergency room 7 days post-delivery because he was sleeping excessively, having few wet and dirty diapers, and was too weak to latch. Samuel was admitted to the children's hospital because he was dehydrated and had an elevated serum bilirubin level. Samuel was started on phototherapy and supplemental feedings. Unfortunately, among healthy LPIs, the ability to breastfeed at discharge and to continue successful breastfeeding at home are persistent independent risk factors for neonatal readmission to hospital due to feeding difficulties [45, 46]. In these circumstances, parents often encounter difficulties in maintaining milk supply [3, 47–49] and milk transfer [13]. These difficulties are most prominent during the first few weeks after birth [12] and contribute to rehospitalizations [4, 50–52] and parental decisions to discontinue breastfeeding [12, 53]. Continued assessment and intervention beyond the first 1–2 days post-hospital discharge by a HCP remains important for LPI health and breastfeeding success. Consideration should include:

7.6.1   Maternal Milk Supply

Mothers of LPIs may have compromised milk supply or delay in mature milk production from medical issues that contributed to early birth, such as gestational diabetes, gestational hypertension, preeclampsia, multiple fetuses, preterm labor, cesarean section, blood loss, and infection [7, 54]. The LPI may also provide inadequate breast stimulation and removal of milk from the breasts, resulting in decreased production of milk from ineffective suckling attempts [12]. After the initial direct breastfeeding session or hand expression, hand or pump expression alone or in conjunction with direct feedings should occur approximately every 2–3 h to sustain or maintain milk supply [25, 55–57]. Acquisition of an electric pump can provide valuable support to mothers by ensuring adequate breast emptying, facilitating the establishment of maternal milk supply, and allaying fears of milk insufficiency [14, 43, 58, 59]. In the United States and Canada, access to breast pumps for some mothers has been financially problematic; however, initiatives to provide electric pump access through private insurance companies and government subsidized programs have enabled electric pump utilization for a larger number of women [14]. The US Special Supplemental Nutrition Program for Women, Infants, and Children program offers peer support counselors to aid mothers in the navigation of breastfeeding in the home and community environments and includes education for proper use of electric pumps [14]. In cases where early and frequent breast stimulation, expression, and emptying are inadequate, milk supply is compromised [12]. This increases the risk of shorter breastfeeding durations and loss of breastfeeding exclusivity for LPIs in the first 6 months of life [60]. Consequently, the rate of breastfeeding exclusivity and duration for LPIs are significantly less than their term counterparts [4, 60]. Mothers should be cautioned from weaning manual or pumped breast expression too rapidly to ensure breast emptying and the establishment of milk supply [3, 13].

Breastfeeding rates for the LPI drop dramatically within 4–10 weeks following birth. Hackman and colleagues [53] conducted a large study with mothers, 116 of whom delivered LPIs. The researchers found several reasons mothers of LPIs discontinued breastfeeding within 1 month after birth. These were related to mothers' reports of not having enough milk to feed their infant and latching difficulties. This timeline is similar with the work of Kair and Colaizy [58], wherein mothers of LPIs discontinued breastfeeding within 10 weeks of giving birth due to insufficient milk supply, hence the need for providers to continue offering breastfeeding support and strategies for maintaining or increasing milk supply. Positive variables that support mothers of LPIs to breastfeed beyond 1 month after birth include attendance at a prenatal breastfeeding class, education beyond high school, deciding to breastfeed within pregnancy, and planning to breastfeed for at least 6 months [53, 58]. Some variables that increased the mother's risk of a shorter breastfeeding duration include smoking, single-parent status, and a high pre-pregnancy basal metabolic rate [53, 58].

7.6.2   Insufficient Milk Transfer and Supplemental Feeding

When feeding attempts are unsuccessful, supplementation of breastfeeding sessions with expressed human milk, donor pasteurized human milk, or formula may be necessary [3]. If insufficient milk transfer is expected or confirmed, breast compressions during infant suckling and the use of an ultrathin silicone nipple shield should be considered for low-resource settings [3, 12]. Nipple shields can be filled with expressed human milk or formula to encourage a nutritive suck at the breast [8]. Nipple shields help the infant to achieve vacuum pressure required for extraction of milk from the breast [38, 61, 62]. Additional approaches include the use of droppers, syringes, spoons, cup, feeding tubes, and bottles that can be filled with human milk or formula and put in the side of the infant's mouth while latching at the breast to provide nutrients, supplementation, and offer breast stimulation for increasing milk supply [3, 8, 12, 21]. Supplementation of 5–10 ml per feeding on the first day of life and 10–30 ml per feeding each subsequent day of hospitalization can protect infant health and hydration.

There are several considerations when choosing bottle feeding as a supplemental feeding method. The use of bottle feeding may be challenging for the LPI due to difficulties with suck, swallow, and breath coordination and milk flowing too quickly for the infant to control [61]. Infants require paced feedings with pauses between sucks and swallows and tilting the bottle only slightly so it is aligned with the baby's mouth [31, 35]. LPIs also require slow-flow nipples with slow volumes extracted from each suck on the bottle to decrease choking and gagging, and to increase suck, swallow, and breathe coordination [12, 35]. Parents should be taught to wait for their infant to present with a wide-open mouth before proceeding with a feed [10]. As with breastfeeds, parents should be supported to not focus on volume-driven bottle-feeds providing a slow-paced relaxed feeding environment [34, 35].

Regardless of the chosen supplementation feeding method, parents should be taught to provide supplemental feedings when infants are sleepy and fatigued while reserving more alert times for direct breastfeeding sessions [3]. In addition, LPIs tire easily with all types of feeding, and parents should be taught the previously mentioned disengagement cues, as well as signs of exhaustion including fussiness, falling asleep while feeding, turning away from the bottle, and pushing the bottle out of the mouth [10, 30, 63]. The utilization of supplemental feeding methods and therapeutic feeding devices should be based upon the clinical situation, maternal preference, and the experience of the provider who is assisting the mother [3].

7.6.3   Transitioning to the Breast feeding

Transitioning to exclusive breastfeeding may take several weeks. Parents need to know that exclusive breastfeeding is a developmental process that occurs as the LPI matures and develops. All feeding attempts should be recognized and acknowledged by HCPs with the parents and caregivers. Parents should be encouraged to continue regular skin-to-skin contact with their infants to promote bonding and earlier establishment and sustainability of breastfeeding [19, 63, 64]. Infants need to lick and suckle at the breast to release the milk hormones oxytocin and prolactin and be encouraged to latch at the breast with every feed or several times a day even for short durations [19]. Mothers should continue to express milk and supplement their LPI until the infant has adequate output and weight gain [63]. Expressed milk on the nipple can be used to entice infants to suckle and latch. With a delay in letdown of the milk reflex, some infants become frustrated when milk is not readily available as with the cup or bottle [65]. Providers can support mothers to express breastmilk to stimulate the letdown reflex before placing baby on the breast. Mothers should maintain the infant in a flexed midline position and observe for a good latch [31, 34]. Upon latching, the infant should be calm and not appear to struggle to re-latch or "fight" with the breast [32]. The infant should suck continuously and rhythmically with frequent swallowing for greater then 15 min to ensure an effective feeding session [65]. Observing infant cues, initiating feeds when alert and focused, and recognition of infant disorganization will enable successful transition to the breast and a pleasant feeding experience for all [32].

7.7   Tailored Maternal Education and Breastfeeding Support

7.7.1   Thermoregulation

LPIs have less ability than full-term infants to regulate their body temperatures due to limited amounts of white adipose tissue, ineffective heat generation from brown adipose tissue, and a susceptibility to lose heat because of a larger ratio of weight to surface area [41]. Infants will feed more effectively if thermoregulation is maintained by placing the infant naked on the mother's chest during a feed reducing hypothermia or hyperthermia [28]. When not participating in breastfeeding sessions, hypothermia can be avoided by urging frequent skin-to-skin contact sessions and by double wrapping the infant with clothing, blankets, and a hat [3].

7.7.2   Hypoglycemia

LPIs are at an increased risk for hypoglycemia after birth due to immature metabolic pathways, a higher metabolic rate, and limited energy stores [12, 41]. Manifestations encompass symptoms common to ill neonates including shaking, trembling, or seizures; cyanosis; respiratory distress or apnea episodes; and weak cry, lethargy, or sleepiness [66]. Continuation of breastfeeding every 2–3 h, supplemental feedings, or intravenous dextrose may be indicated for low blood glucose levels and weight loss [3]. There is a lack of general agreement for predicting blood glucose levels which may result in adverse neurologic outcomes for infants [66].

7.7.3   Hyperbilirubinemia or Jaundice

LPIs are particularly at risk for "lack of breastmilk" jaundice caused by infrequent or ineffective breastfeeding [12]. As already discussed, LPIs experience more feeding difficulties leading to lack of milk transfer and/or delays in milk production. This low caloric intake combined with limitations in bilirubin metabolism and transport, leads to an increase of bilirubin in the blood [12]. Jaundice can interfere with feeding efforts as LPIs tire easily and may not be interested in feeding yet require adequate milk transfer to assist with bilirubin conjugation [12]. Thus, LPIs should be monitored closely for inadequate milk intake and rising bilirubin levels that could progress to "lack of breastmilk jaundice," decreased number of stools, and increased risk for excessive and prolonged jaundice [3, 12]. LPIs require adequate milk transfer through regular feedings to assist with conjugation of bilirubin, such as 10–12 feeds within 24 h, adequate fecal output, or phototherapy if serum bilirubin levels are above safe parameters [67]. Parents can be also taught to monitor increased signs and symptoms of jaundice:

Signs and symptoms of jaundice [67]:

- Yellowing of the skin beginning with the head and sclera of the eyes progressing caudally to the chest and umbilical area
- Decreased urine and fecal output
- Difficulty rousing for feedings or sleepiness during feeds
- Weight loss
- Dehydration
- Decreased muscle tone

Community HCPs should offer frequent breastfeeding support for LPIs in the first week following delivery and hospital discharge and provide continued monitoring of transcutaneous and/or serum bilirubin levels as this is the time frame when LPIs are most at risk for hyperbilirubinemia [46, 68, 69].

7.7.4 Home Feeding Environment

Some LPIs are unable to feed successfully unless the home environment is calm with few distractions and limited noise [10, 34]. Feeding times should remain quiet, so LPIs can focus on one activity at a time and experience feeding exclusively. LPIs may benefit from increased stimulation like singing, rocking, and skin massages at nonfeeding times for enhanced growth and development [8, 10, 63]. In addition, LPIs prefer a consistent approach to feeding from caregivers, whether by bottle with expressed human milk or formula [35]. It is appropriate to discuss the feeding environment with all caregivers who will feed the LPI.

7.7.5 Return to Work Challenges

Some mothers return to work in the early postpartum period without sufficient government assisted maternity leaves. After examining global literature for promoting breastfeeding practices within the workplace, authors relayed the need for institutional policies that support breastfeeding in the work site [70, 71] and government legislation to extend job-protected maternity leaves [70]. Returning to work without a sufficient maternity leave can become a barrier for maintaining milk supply as mothers return to work. Women may need use of a breast pump for removal of breast milk to maintain their milk supply. Ideally, working mothers should have access to pumps while separated from their infants and breastfeed their infants before work, during the lunch hour (when possible), after work, and before sleeping [70, 71]. Other suggestions for improving breastfeeding continuation among working mothers include educating mothers and employers about benefits of accommodating breastfeeding in the workplace, supporting mothers in developing realistic goals, building confidence and motivation to continue feeding upon return to work, and a supportive environment for feeding the infant while at work from peers and employers [70, 71]. Historically, workplaces have not provided mothers with appropriate break times or areas to both breastfeed and to use a breast pump and store breastmilk [70–72]. Oftentimes, mothers resorted to pumping in bathrooms, and many mothers ceased breastfeeding due to workplace breastfeeding conflicts. The Affordable Care Act [73] introduced an amendment within the United States to address workplace breastfeeding barriers for mothers and included provisions to allow for reasonable break times and a private area, other than a restroom, for mothers to express milk for up to 1 year postpartum [73]. Despite these legal provisions, Kozhimannil and colleagues [72] recently explored women's workplace breastfeeding provisions and found that only 40% of the American national sample of 2400 mothers had access to both adequate break times and a private area for milk expression. Women with the proper legal provisions were 2.3 times (95% CI, 1.03–4.95) as likely to continue exclusive breastfeeding at 6 months postpartum. Thus, non-breastfeeding-friendly workplace environments remain a concern for mothers globally and contribute to early breastfeeding cessation.

7.8   Hospital Discharge Planning and Home Follow-Up

Sara was discharged home with feeding instructions that were appropriate for a normal-term infant but insufficient for Samuel. Who was a LPI additionally, Sara was not offered early home visits or follow-up from HCPs that could have prevented Samuel's extreme weight loss, dehydration, jaundice, and hospital readmission. When planning for discharge from the postpartum hospital stay, the infant's physiologic stability, feeding regimen, and home follow-up plan should be thoroughly assessed and confirmed, with in-depth education and instruction provided to parents in both written and verbal forms [3, 44]. This plan should address interventions to protect the medical vulnerabilities of LPIs and consider social and environmental risk factors for the family, family support and dynamics [5, 13, 14]. Weight loss should be assessed prior to discharge and should ideally be no more than 7% of the infant's birth weight. However, discharge may still be appropriate if supplementation strategies ensure adequate milk intake and the infant's weight loss is trending toward stabilization or weight gain [3].

The discharge feeding plan should be continually monitored by HCPs in the weeks after birth to address ongoing concerns with milk transfer, milk intake, and weight loss [3]. Ongoing assessment, teaching, and intervention with supplemental feedings and therapeutic feeding devices are often necessary in the weeks after hospital discharge [3]. The community HCP should reassess the utility and effectiveness of these devices and supplementation methods with parents to ensure adequate milk intake and family comfort with the feeding plan during the weeks after discharge. Immature, inconsistent, and unsystematic feeding behaviors, which present as subtle feeding cues, sleepiness or fatiguing easily during feedings, as well as oromotor dysfunction may persist in LPIs until 40 weeks of conceptual age [3, 47–49], a in same instances beyond this time. Parents require support and encouragement from experienced HCPs with lactation expertise.

The mother's emotional state and fatigue, along with degree of nipple trauma and pain, could serve as indicators for the effectiveness of the home feeding plan [3]. The HCP should observe a direct feeding session with the mother and infant to address any problems with latch, suck, and swallow patterns. The feeding plan may need revision based upon family support needs and feasibility of maintaining the original feeding plan. Weekly weight checks with a HCP should continue until the LPI is gaining weight at an average of 20–30 g/day and the family has an established level of comfort with the infant's feeding patterns and schedule [3].

While in the hospital, Sara voiced concerns about Samuel's lack of energy and fatigue with feedings. Those concerns likely contributed to confusion and anxiety at home for Sara when trying to determine if baby Samuel was nursing properly and maintaining a healthy weight. The infant and mother should be assessed for signs of wellness or distress, anxiety, and fatigue [3, 5, 13, 44, 74]. Parental anxiety over infant health is an important consideration in the LPI's adjustment from the hospital to the home environment, and supportive care from experienced and qualified HCPs is instrumental in developing parental confidence about safe and appropriate care of the infant at home [75]. Anxiety and stress in mothers caring for an LPI can impact breastfeeding duration rates and maternal milk supply due to physiological and behavioral processes that affect the letdown reflex and other physiological mechanisms [76]. Additionally, breastfeeding difficulties persist due to lack of support, isolation, and maternal fatigue [46, 77–80]. The complexity of supplemental feeding, along with the time required to manage various feeding methods, may be overwhelming for a mother who is likely already fatigued and is recovering from delivery. For most parents, confidence in caring for their LPI improved after approximately 1 month of seeing the infant progress and gain weight [81]. Some parents took up to 1 year to feel comfortable with caring for their infants [78, 82, 83].

Providers should also assess parental support and coping mechanisms [3, 5, 44]. Positive, encouraging, early support from providers and peer counselors, increases the parent's confidence in caring for their LPI and can increase breastfeeding duration [14, 23, 75, 84]. Parents appreciate reinforcement about feeding positions and responding to cues [23, 35, 48], consistent advice from caregivers [13], education about the LPI's unique physical challenges [79, 84], recognizing feeding distress [13], and anticipatory guidance of expectations in the first few weeks upon discharge home [58, 77, 85–87]. Furthermore, specialized knowledge of LPIs by HCPs is essential in providing appropriate comprehensive care [87–90]. HCPs working in the community require knowledge of effective and evidence-based low-resource interventions to reduce variability in care and meet community specific needs [87]. In a recent study on the experience of caring for LPIs in the community, community health nurses relayed difficulty in establishing successful breastfeeding routines with LPIs due to lack of healthcare resources for families, a shortage of evidence informed guidelines, and inconsistent practices among nurses [62, 87]. Available resources for HCPs caring for LPIs include breastfeeding guidelines for optimal health, growth, and brain development [2, 3, 67]. LPIs may require further support from community LCs. Consultation with a qualified LC should be considered as substantial and relevant, and referral should occur soon after arriving home [3, 9, 46, 54, 69]. Some lactation services are privately funded requiring parents pay consultation fees on their own. Other LCs work for public health agencies or healthcare clinics and provide subsidized or free support to families caring for LPIs. Most midwives provide lactation support instead of a LC, particularly in low-resource settings. Overall formation of multidisciplinary teams has also been found to contribute to better service provision for families with lactation and other health issues [91].

7.9   Clinical Case Study Wrap-Up

After readmission to the hospital, Sara was visited by a HCP twice per day to evaluate Samuel's feeding sessions. Although Samuel appeared to have a adequate latch, suck, and swallow pattern, lack of dirty diapers confirmed that his milk transfer and volume intake remained inadequate for proper weight gain. The HCP demonstrated use of an electric pump for milk removal and cup-feeding supplementation to ensure proper milk volume intake. After discharge home from the hospital the second time, a community health nurse visited Sara and Samuel and determined that Samuel was feeding well with an appropriate feeding plan for the family in the home environment. Sara received regular home visits from the community health nurse and visited the primary provider weekly until Samuel no longer required cup-feeding supplementation to maintain weight gain for proper growth and development. Sara gained confidence with breastfeeding after the rehospitalization and continued to breastfeed Samuel for his first year of life.

Conclusion
Successful breastfeeding of LPIs is complex and presents multiple challenges for parents and HCPs. Feeding assessments should be conducted early and often,

considering the physiological stability of the infant and feeding difficulties specific to LPIs. Early and consistent parental education specific to the comfort level of the family is essential to instill parental confidence in infant care, adherence to the feeding plan, and ensure successful exclusive breastfeeding. Furthermore, a comprehensive feeding plan that is well-developed and communicated to parents and all members of the healthcare team within the hosptial and community environments, helps to facilitate successful and exclusive breastfeeding of LPIs.

References

1. U.S. Department of Health and Human Services. Executive summary: the surgeon general's call to action to support breastfeeding. Washington, DC: U.S. Department of Health and Human Services; 2011.
2. Eidelman A, Schanler R, Johnston M, et al. American Academy of Pediatrics section on breast-feeding. Breastfeeding and the use of human milk. Pediatrics. 2012;129(3):e827–41.
3. Boies E, Vaucher Y, The Academy of Breastfeeding Medicine. ABM clinical protocol #10: breastfeeding the late preterm (34–36 6/7 weeks of gestation) and early term infants (37–38 6/7 week of gestation), second revision. Breastfeed Med. 2016;11(10):494–500.
4. Goyal NK, Attanasio LB, Kozhimannil KB. Hospital care and early breastfeeding outcomes among late preterm, early-term, and term infants. Birth. 2014;41(4):330–7.
5. Vohr B, et al. Impact of a transitional home program on rehospitalization rates of preterm infants. J Pediatr. 2017;181(e81):86–92.
6. Pea S. Developmental outcomes of late preterm infants from infancy to kindergarten. Pediatrics. 2016;138(2):e20153496.
7. Meier P, Patel A, Wright K, Engstrom J. Management of breastfeeding during and after the maternity hospitalization for late preterm infants. Clin Perinatol. 2013;40(4):689–705.
8. Walker M. Breastfeeding management for the late preterm infant: Practical interventions for "Little Imposters". Clin Lactat. 2010;1(1):22–6.
9. Mally PV, Bailey S, Hendricks-Munoz KD. Clinical issues in the management of late preterm infants. Curr Probl Pediatr Adolesc Health Care. 2010;40:218–33.
10. Thompson DG. Focusing on feeding skills evaluating inadequate weight gain in late preterm infants. Infant Child Adolesc Nutr. 2010;2(3):147–51.
11. Eidelman A. The challenge of breastfeeding the late preterm and the early-term infant. Breastfeed Med. 2016;11(3):99.
12. Meier P, Furman L, Degenhardt M. Increased lactation risk for late preterm infants and moth-ers: evidence and management strategies to protect breastfeeding. J Midwifery Womens Health. 2007;52:579–87.
13. Premji S, Currie G, Reilly S, Dosani A, Oliver LM, Lodha AK, Young M. A qualitative study: mothers of late preterm infants relate their experiences of community-based care. PLoS One. 2017;12(3):30174419.
14. Bennett C, Galloway C, Grassley J. Education for WIC peer counselors about breastfeeding the late preterm infant. J Nutr Educ Behav. 2018;50(2):198–202.e1.
15. World Health Organization. Baby-friendly hospital initiative: revised, updated and expanded for integrated care. Geneva: WHO; 2009. http://www.ncbi.nlm.nih.gov/books/NBK153495/. Accessed 2017 August 30
16. Munn A, Newman SD, Mueller M, Phillips SM, Taylor SN. The impact in the United States of the Baby-Friendly Hospital Initiative on early infant health and breastfeeding outcomes. Breastfeed Med. 2016;11(5):222–30.

17. Baby-Friendly USA. The ten steps to successful breastfeeding. New York, NY: Baby-Friendly USA; 2012. Available from: https://www.babyfriendlyusa.org/about-us/baby-friendly-hospital-initiative/the-ten-steps

18. Moore ER, Anderson GC, Bergman N, Dowswell T. Early skin-to-skin contact for mothers and their healthy newborn infants. Cochrane Database Syst Rev. 2012;2012(5):Art. No.: CD003519.

19. Phillips R. Uninterrupted skin-to-skin contact immediately after birth. Newborn Infant Nurs Rev. 2013;13(2):67–72. Available from: www.medscape.com. Accessed 23 Jul 2016

20. Widestrom A, Wahlberg V, Matthiesen A. Short-term effects of early suckling and touch of the nipple on maternal behaviour. Early Hum Dev. 1990;21:153–63.

21. Briere C-E, Lucas R, McGrath J, Lussier M, Brownell E. Establishing breastfeeding with the late preterm infant in the NICU. J Obstet Gynecol Neonatal Nurs. 2015;44:102–13.

22. Meier P, Patel AL, Bigger HR, Rossman B, Engstrom AL. Supporting breastfeeding in the neonatal intensive care unit: Rush mother's milk club as a case study of evidence-based care. Pediatr Clin N Am. 2013;60:209–26. https://doi.org/10.1016/j.pcl.2012.10.007. Accessed 12 Jul 2017

23. Gianni M, Bezze E, Sannino P, Stori E, Plevani L, Roggero P, et al. Facilitators and barriers of breastfeeding late preterm infants according to mothers' experiences. BMC Pediatr. 2016;16(1):179.

24. Parker LA, Sullivan S, Krueger C, et al. Effect of early milk expression on milk volume and timing of lactogenesis stage II among mothers of very low birthweight infants: a pilot study. J Perinatol. 2012;32:205–9.

25. Morton J, Hall JY, Wong RJ, Thairu L, Benitz WE, Rhine WD. Combining hand techniques with electric pumping increases milk production in mothers of preterm infants. J Perinatol. 2009;29(11):757–64.

26. Flacking R, Ewald U, Wallin L. Positive effect of kangaroo mother care on long-term breast-feeding in very preterm infants. J Obstet Gynecol Neonatal Nurs. 2011;40(2):190–7.

27. Nyqvist KH, Häggkvist A-P, Hansen MN, Kylberg E, Frandsen AL, Maastrup R, et al. Expansion of the Baby-Friendly Hospital initiative ten steps to successful breastfeeding into neonatal intensive care: expert group recommendations. J Hum Lact. 2013;29(3):300–9.

28. Niela-Vilen H, Axelin A, Salantera S, Lehtonen L, Tammela O, Salmelin R, Latva R. Early physical contact between a mother and her NICU-infant in two university hospitals in Finland. Midwifery. 2013;29(12):1321–30.

29. Neu J. Gastrointestinal maturation and feeding. Semin Perinatol. 2006;30(2):77–80.

30. Thoyre S, Shaker C, Pridham K. The early feeding skills assessment for preterm infants. Neonatal Netw. 2005;24(3):7–16.

31. Shaker C. Nipple feeding preterm infants: an individualized, developmentally supportive approach. Neonatal Netw. 1999;18(3):15–22.

32. White CSM, Bryan A. Using evidence to educate birthing center nursing staff: about infant states, cues, and behaviors. Am J Matern Child Nurs. 2002;27(5):294–8.

33. Browne JV, Ross ES. Eating as a neurodevelopmental process for high-risk newborns. Clin Perinatol. 2011;38(4):731–43.

34. Shaker C. Reading the feeding. ASHA Leader. 2013;18:42–7.

35. Shaker C. Cue-based Co-regulated feeding in the neonatal intensive care unit: supporting parents in learning to feed their preterm infant. Newborn Infant Nurs News. 2013;13:51–5.

36. Baker B. Evidence-based practice to improve outcomes for late preterm infants. J Obstet Gynecol Neonatal Nurs. 2015;44(1):127–34.

37. Shaker C. Cue-based feeding in the NICU: using the infant's communication as a guide. Neonatal Netw. 2013;32(6):404–8.

38. Fucile S, McFarland DH, Gisel EG, Lau C. Oral and nonoral sensorimotor interventions facilitate suck–swallow–respiration functions and their coordination in preterm infants. Early Hum Dev. 2012;88(6):345–50.

39. Jensen D, Wallace S, Kelsay PA. Breastfeeding charting system and documentation tool. J Obstet Gynecol Neonatal Nurs. 1994;23:27–32.

40. Altunas N, Kocak M, Akkurt S, Razi H, Kislal M. LATCH scores and milk intake in preterm and term infants: a prospective comparative Study. Breastfeed Med. 2015;10(2):96–101.
41. Engle WA, Tomashek KM, Wallman C, The Committee on Fetus and Newborn. "Late-preterm" infants: a population at risk. Pediatrics. 2007;120(6):1390–401.
42. Lau C. Development of suck and swallow mechanisms in infants. Ann Nutr Metab. 2015;66(Suppl. 5):7–14.
43. Hallowell S, Spatz D. The relationship of brain development and breastfeeding in the late preterm infant. J Pediatr Nurs. 2012;27:154–62.
44. Phillips R, Goldstein M, Houghland K, Nandyal R, Pizzica A, Santa-Donato A, Staebler A, Stark A, Treiger T. Yost, on behalf of The National Perinatal Association. Multidisciplinary guidelines for the care of late preterm infants. J Perinatol. 2013;33(Suppl 2): S5–S22.
45. Tomashek KM, Shapiro-Mendoza CK, Davidoff MJ, Petrini JR. Differences in mortality between late-preterm and term singleton infants in the United States, 1995–2002. J Pediatr. 2007;151:450–6.
46. Young P, Korgenski K, Buchi KF. Early readmission of newborns in a large health care system. Pediatrics. 2013;131(5):e1538–44.
47. DeMauro SBPP, Medoff-Cooper B, Posencheg M, Abbasi S. Postdischarge feeding patterns in early- and late-preterm infants. Clin Pediatr. 2011;50(10):957–62.
48. Medoff-Cooper B, Bilker W, Kaplan J. Sucking behavior as a function of gestational age: a cross-sectional study. Infant Behav Dev. 2001;24(1):83–94.
49. Wang M, Doer D, Fleming M, Catlin E. Clinical outcomes of near-term infants. Pediatrics. 2004;114(2):372–6.
50. Escobar GJ, Clark RH, Greene JD. Short-term outcomes of infants born at 35 and 36 weeks gestation: we need to ask more questions. Semin Perinatol. 2006;30(1):28–33.
51. Jain S, Cheng J. Emergency department visits and rehospitalizations in late preterm infants. Clin Perinatol. 2006;33(4):935–45.
52. Ray KN, Lorch SA. Hospitalization of early preterm, late preterm, and term infants during the first year of life by gestational age. Pediatrics. 2013;3(3):194.
53. Hackman NM, et al. Reduced breastfeeding rates in firstborn late preterm and early term infants. Breastfeed Med. 2016;11:119–25.
54. Adamkin DH. Feeding problems in the late preterm infant. Clin Perinatol. 2006;33(4): 831–7.
55. Hill PD, Aldag JC, Chatterton RT. Initiation and frequency of pumping and milk production in mothers of non-nursing preterm infants. J Hum Lact. 2001;17:9–13.
56. Yilmaz G, Caylan N, Karacan CD, Bodur İ, Gokcay G. Effect of cup feeding and bottle feeding on breastfeeding in late preterm infants a randomized controlled study. J Hum Lact. 2014;17:174–9.
57. Ohyama M, Watabe H, Hayasaka Y. Manual expression and electric breast pumping in the first 48 h after delivery. Pediatr Int. 2010;52(1):39 43.
58. Kair L, Colaizy T. Breastfeeding continuation among late preterm infants: barriers, facilitators, and any association with NICU admission. Hosp Pediatr. 2016;5:261–8.
59. Rasmussen K, Geraghty S. The quiet revolution: breastfeeding transformed with the use of breast pumps. Am J Public Health. 2011;101(8):1356–9.
60. Ayton J, Hansen E, Quinn S, Nelson M. Factors associated with initiation and exclusive breast-feeding at hospital discharge: late preterm compared to 37 week gestation mother and infant cohort. Int Breastfeed J. 2012;7(1):16.
61. Hurst N. Assessing and facilitating milk transfer during breastfeeding for the premature infant. Newborn Infant Nurs Rev. 2005;5(1):19–26.
62. Meier PP, Brown LP, Hurst NM, Spatz DL, Engstrom JL, Borucki LC, Krouse AM. Nipple shields for preterm infants: effect on milk transfer and duration of breastfeeding. J Hum Lact. 2000;16(2):106–14.
63. Hubbard E, Stellwagen L, Wolf A. The late preterm infant: a little baby with big needs. Contemp Pediatr. 2007;24(11):51–9.

64. Scher MS, Ludington-Hoe S, Kaffashi F, Johnson MW, Holditch-Davis D, Loparo KA. Neurophysiologic assessment of brain maturation after an 8-week trial of skin-to-skin contact on preterm infants. Clin Neurophysiol. 2009;120(10):1812–8.
65. Lubbe W. Clinicians guide for cue-based transition to oral feeding in preterm infants: an easy-to-use clinical guide. J Eval Clin Pract. 2017;24:80–8. https://doi.org/10.1111/jep.12721.
66. Adamkin DH, Committee on Fetus and Newborn. Clinical report-postnatal glucose homeostasis in late-preterm and term infants. Pediatrics. 2011;127(3):575–9.
67. Smith JR, Donze A, Schuller L. An evidence-based review of hyperbilirubinemia in the late preterm infant, with implications for practice: management, follow-up and breastfeeding support. Neonatal Netw. 2006;26(6):395–405.
68. Dosani A, Currie G. Supporting public health nurses with breastfeeding interventions for late preterm infants. Austin Pediatr. 2017;4(2):1–13.
69. Watchko JF. Hyperbilirubinemia and bilirubin toxicity in the late preterm infant. Clin Perinatol. 2006;33(4):839–52.
70. Hirani SA, Karmaliani R. Evidence based workplace interventions to promote breastfeeding practices among Pakistani working mothers. Women Birth. 2013;26(1):10–6.
71. Hirani SA, Premji SS. Mother's employment and breastfeeding continuation: global and Pakistani perspectives from the literature. Neonatal Pediatr Child Health Nurs. 2009;12(2):18–24.
72. Kozhimannil KB, Jou J, Gjerdingen DK, McGovern PM. Access to workplace accommodations to support breastfeeding after passage of the affordable care act. Womens Health Issues. 2016;26(1):6–13.
73. U.S. Department of Health and Human Services Affordable care act expands prevention coverage for women's health and well-being. Available from: www.hrsa.gov/womensguidelines. Accessed 10 July, 2014. 2010.
74. Tully K, Holditch-Davis D, Silva S, Brandon D. The relationship between infant feeding outcomes and maternal emotional well-being among mothers of late preterm and term infants: a secondary, exploratory analysis. Adv Neonatal Care. 2017;17(1):65–75.
75. Adama EA, Bayes S, Sundin D. Parents' experiences of caring for preterm infants after discharge from neonatal intensive care unit: a meta-synthesis of the literature. J Neonatal Nurs. 2016;22(1):27–51.
76. Zanardo V, Gabrieli C, Straface G, Savio F, Soldera G. The interaction of personality profile and lactation differs between mothers of late preterm and term neonates. J Matern Fetal Neonat Med. 2017;30(8):927–32.
77. Dosani A, Hemraj J, Premji SS, Currie G, Reilly SM, Lodha AK, Young M, Hall M. Breastfeeding the late preterm infant: experiences of mothers and perceptions of public health nurses. Int Breastfeed J. 2017;12:23.
78. Howe TH, Sheu CF, Wang TN, Hsu YW. Parenting stress in families with very low birth weight preterm infants in early infancy. Res Dev Disabil. 2014;35(7):1748–56.
79. Kair LR, Flaherman VJ, Newby KA, Colaizy T. The experience of breastfeeding the late preterm infant: a qualitative study. Breastfeed Med. 2015;10(2):102–6.
80. Radtke Demerici J, Happ MB, Bogen DL, Albrecht SA, Cohen SM. Weighing worth against uncertain work: the interplay of exhaustion, ambiguity, hope and disappointment in mothers breastfeeding late preterm infants. Matern Child Nutr. 2015;11(1):59–72.
81. Griffin JB, Pickler RH. Hospital-to-home transition of mothers of preterm infants. Am J Matern Child Nurs. 2011;36(4):252–7.
82. Jackson K, Ternestedt BM, Schollin J. From alienation to familiarity: Experiences of mothers and fathers of preterm infants. J Adv Nurs. 2003;43:120–9.
83. Phillips-Pula L, Pickler R, McGrath JM, Brown LF, Dusing SC. Caring for a preterm infant at home: a mother's perspective. J Perinat Neonat Nurs. 2013;27(4):335–44.
84. Olson BH, Haider SJVL, Bolton TA, Gold JG. A quasi-experimental evaluation of a breastfeeding support program for low income women in Michigan. Matern Child Health J. 2010;14(1):86–93.

85. Boykova M. Transition from hospital to home in parents of preterm infants. J Perinat Neonat Nurs. 2016;30(4):327–248.
86. Quinn JM, Sparks M, Gephart SM. Discharge criteria for the late preterm infant: a review of the literature. Adv Neonatal Care. 2017;17(5):362–71.
87. Currie G, Dosani A, Premji S, Reilly S, Lodha A, Young M, et al. Caring for late preterm infants: public health nurses' experiences. BMC Nurs. 2018;17:16.
88. Ravn IH, Smith L, Smeby NA, Kynoe NM, Sandvik L, Bunch EH, Lindemann R. Effects of early mother–infant intervention on outcomes in mothers and moderately and late preterm infants at age 1 year: a randomized controlled trial. Infant Behav Dev. 2012;35(1):36–47.
89. Boykova M, Kenner C. Transition from hospital to home for parents of preterm infants. J Perinat Neonat Nurs. 2012;26(1):81–7.
90. Russell SA, Rabe H, Abbott J, Gyte G, Duley L, et al. Parents' views on care of their very premature babies in neonatal intensive care units: a qualitative study. BMC Pediatr. 2014;14(230):501.
91. Association of Women's Health Obstetrical and Neonatal Nurses. Assessment and care of the late preterm infant: Evidence-based clinical practice guidelines. Washington, DC: Association of Women's Health Obstetrical and Neonatal Nurses; 2010.

How Do You Wean a Late Preterm Infant Off Supplements: You Mean I Have to Suck Feed?

8

Jennifer Marandola and Karen Lasby

8.1 Introduction

In hospital, treatment recommendations for the late preterm infant tend to focus on glucose and temperature instability, respiratory distress, and apnea and bradycardia. Typically, these are resolved within the first 48 h. In the community however, there are challenges of caring for the late preterm infant that may persist for the first several weeks. Among these challenges is the continued poor feeding skills of the late preterm infant and the continued efforts of the parents to progress toward exclusive breastfeeding. Many healthcare professionals still focus on the "normalization" of the LPIs and often portray a false image of what transition to community will be like for the mother and her infant [1]. It is our job as healthcare providers to offer continued support and strategies to the parents as the newborn continues to develop. When it comes to breastfeeding late preterm infants, one of two things can happen at hospital discharge: either the infant was alert and feeding well post-birth and deteriorates day 2 or 3, or they have yet to have a good feed at the breast prior to discharged. Many hospitals have yet to have a minimum 48-h discharge policy with this population which can often leave parents to deal with the continuing challenges on their own with limited support. Early hospital discharge almost always assumes early community follow-up, and this is not always the case; thus, parent education is critical to ensuring successful transition to exclusive breastfeeding.

There is a large amount of literature focusing on the feeding difficulties experienced by early preterm infants; however, the incidence of feeding difficulties in late

J. Marandola (✉)

volet Jeunesse/Santé-Publique, Centre intégré universitaire de santé et de services sociaux de l'Ouest-de-l'île-de-Montréal,
Montréal, QC, Canada

K. Lasby
Neonatal Transition Team, Postpartum Services, Calgary, AB, Canada
e-mail: karen.lasby@albertahealthservices.ca

© Springer International Publishing AG, part of Springer Nature 2019
S. S. Premji (ed.), *Late Preterm Infants*, https://doi.org/10.1007/978-3-319-94352-7_8

preterm infants is unknown and often underreported [2]. What has come out in recent literature is that late preterm infants have lower exclusive breastfeeding rates than both term and early term infants in part, because families do not receive sufficient and appropriate support in the immediate postpartum period [3]. It has been said that this is due in part to the focus on early discharge from hospital, a period when late preterm infants could be masking poor feeding skills by giving the impression to both healthcare workers and their parents that they are feeding sufficiently; however this impression will change once in the community when larger volumes of milk are required and the immature feeding skills of the late preterm infant cannot meet the demands required [3]. As such, the role of healthcare workers in the community becomes incredibly important for this population. What is equally important is for the public health nurse to provide a plethora of strategies and tools that the new mother can use on her breastfeeding journey as this new mother will quickly learn, her journey is just beginning.

8.2   Role of Healthcare Providers in Anticipatory Guidance

Typically, it can be very beneficial to parents if the facts are presented in a matter-of-fact manner. Inform them that formula supplementation is a temporary solution to a temporary challenge. As the newborn matures and develops stronger feeding skills, we will be able to wean off the supplementation. Encourage them by telling them that this is exactly what formula was invented for, to assist in those situations when breastfeeding is not going as we planned or for whatever reason is not possible. Literature has shown that it can take a late preterm infant a minimum of 6–8 weeks of supplementation before they are able to breastfeed exclusively and efficiently at the breast [3–5].

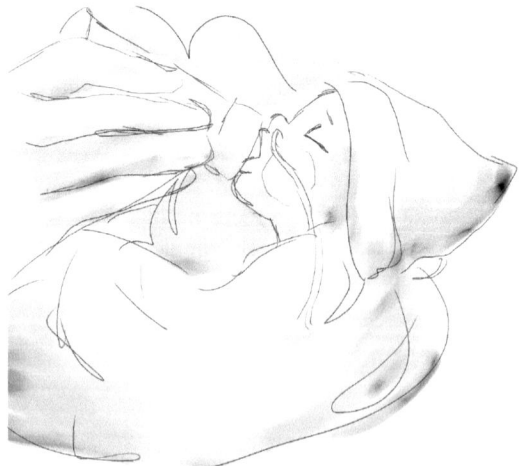

Let them know that it may take 6–8 weeks (sometimes more) for their newborn to progress to exclusive feeds, but in the long-term, this moment is but a stepping stone in their breastfeeding journey. When they look back on this moment, they will see that in the end they spent much more time breastfeeding as they dreamed and very little time in this progressive phase.

So what can we do to help parents and set them off on their journey to exclusive breastfeeding? It should be stated early on what we hope to achieve with a "good feed." In hospital, parents need to learn the importance of a good feed. This should be based on nutritive vs. nonnutritive assessments of how the feed goes. On discharge, they should already know some basics about breastfeeding that will help them in the community:

1. How do I know when my newborn is latched well?
2. How do I know if my newborn is swallowing?
3. How do I know when I need to supplement and when I don't?
4. How do I know how much to give?

These are all questions that should be answered during their hospital stay and continued to be reinforced in the community. In hospital, feeds will be short and frequent (usually on a 2- to 3-h schedule). Healthcare providers tend to emphasize the 2- to 3-h schedule because it is easier to understand and easier to manage. The problem with that is that there is no clear indication as to when parents should stop or change the schedule. As the newborn matures, feeding on demand instincts will become noticeable. If parents do not understand that feeding on demand is normal, they will favor making the newborn wait until the 2 h have passed before feeding again, which can lead to a very unhappy newborn and likewise very unhappy parents. Paying attention to hunger cues and disengagement cue can help parents adjust to this new demand schedule and make for an easier transition to exclusive breastfeeding. Teaching parents these tips without explaining the why or the basics of breastfeeding can cause further challenges for parents down the road.

While scheduling feeds with late preterm infants is important, my advice to new parents typically sounds like this, "If your newborn hasn't woken up by three hours, this is a newborn that you want to wake up to feed because otherwise they'll sleep right through and not necessarily make up for what they have lost. However, if they wake up before the three-hour mark then that's amazing. It tells us that they are developing their feeding cues. You should feed them when they wake up in that case." Due to the difficulty achieving a deep sleep, late preterm infants are not able to achieve a balanced sleep-wake cycle. They will not wake when hungry and will often sleep through feeds, and due to their lack of deep sleep and recuperation in between feeds, the subsequent feeds can often be disorganized and nonnutritive [3]. Teaching the parents this from early on will significantly reduce the time to exclusive breastfeeding.

8.3 Strategies to Consider Before Moving to Supplementation

In community, mothers will often be advised to supplement breastfeeds due to their infants inability to obtain the full nutrients and volume needed from their mother's breast. Infants who were supplemented regularly [1] had longer delay before initiation of breastfeeding, [2] breastfeed less frequently, and [3] had longer hospital stays [6]. As such, it is important that healthcare providers pass on one vital piece of information to parents. Not every feed needs a supplementation; parents need to be aware of how to tell if a supplementation is needed after a feed or not.

Because both breastfeeding and supplementation depend on newborn's hunger cues and disengagement cues, it is important that we emphasize them again.

8.3.1 Hunger Cues

- Sucking on fist.
- Smacking lips.
- Rooting.
- Waking up and restless.
- Crying (late sign).

8.3.2 Disengagement/Stress Cues

- Change is state of alertness.
- Irritable, crying, and falling asleep before adequate feed achieved.
- Change in postural control, tone, or movement patterns.
- Arching, stiffening, flaccid, or limp.
- Changes in physiological stability.
- Tachypnea, apnea, pale, cyanosis, tachycardia, bradycardia, and nasal flaring.
- Lack of synchrony of suck-swallow-breathe reflex.
- Spilling or drooling, gulping, gurgling sounds, multiple swallowing to clear bolus, coughing, and/or choking.

Late preterm infant's hunger cues are often subtle and confusing. A modified demand feeding may be suitable as a temporary measure until the infant reaches behavioral state maturity [7]. In modified demand feeding, if the newborn does not cue in a reasonable time frame from the last feeding, the caregiver assists the newborn to an alert state. Such strategies may include breastmilk drops on the lip, undress infant, change diaper, skin-to-skin, or nonnutritive sucking on finger or soother [7].

Feeding the sleepy low-energy late preterm infant is often challenging. The late preterm infant may start the feed with vigor but quickly lose energy and coordination [8]. Late preterm infants will often take smaller volumes and more frequent feeds due to smaller stomach capacity and early feeding skill. Parents may try feeding as soon as their infant cues hunger. Once their infant shows signs of falling asleep, stop the feed to burp and gently change the infant's diaper, and resume feeding. The short break and diaper change is often enough to arouse the infant to complete another round of feeding. Another strategy is to stop the feed once baby falls asleep as evidenced by closed eyes and limp extremities (rag doll). If the parent is working harder at the feed than the baby, the feeding needs to stop until the infant is engaged again. The parent lies their infant down supine in a safe location without covering with a blanket. While the infant has a short rest, the parent is encouraged to tend to their own needs such as nutrition or rest. The parent should resume feeding once the infant cues again. This strategy reduces parent stress and the tendency to force feed during sleep. This strategy also reinforces cue-based feeding and a positive feeding experience for the newborn. Strategies that may help the sleepy newborn include undress, stroke body/face, and talk to newborn. Avoid noxious stimulation, such as cold cloths.

For newborns with difficulty latching, several techniques exist that can help sustain the latch. Using a syringe to drop some expressed breast milk onto the nipple or in the corner of the newborn's mouth can provide incentive to latch on [9]. Once the baby is latched, placing a few more drops will encourage the newborn to continue the latch and sustained sucking. Breast compressions are also an excellent way to make the newborn more efficient at the breast. When the newborn is latched and sucking well, compressing the breast will help provide extra milk boluses to encourage milk transfer to take place. Healthcare providers should teach parents the importance of breast compressions in these early days, particularly with newborns who are having milk transfer issues.

Another strategy to compensate for weak sucking skills or difficulty sustaining latch is to incorporate a nipple shield [10]. Size 20 is usually a good fit for most late preterm infants though shields are also available in size 16 or 24, if needed. The mother applies the nipple shield by placing a small amount of her milk or water around the inner edge to allow the shield to hold in place. Once the newborn latches, the intraoral vacuum will work to maintain this suction. The mother may also help her infant by expressing some milk into the shield. Once a nipple shield is introduced, mothers should be encouraged to attempt to feed first without the shield and to only apply the shield if the newborn is having difficulty latching to avoid difficulty weaning off the shield later on. A nipple shield might not be necessary at every feed [11].

8.4   Supplementation: Goal of Supplementation

Parents should know that the key to supplementation and weaning off supplementation is that parents and caregivers understand the difference between nutritive and nonnutritive feedings. Families and healthcare professionals are commonly perplexed how to balance the need for sufficient intake to offset hyperbilirubinemia and hypoglycemia and the need to assist the late preterm infant develop breastfeeding competence, cue-based feeding skill, and a positive feeding experience. The demand for increased intake to offset weight loss or hyperbilirubinemia may take precedence over the desired feeding method. For example, supplementation would be provided for late preterm infants with insufficient breastfeeding skill or mothers with low milk supply. Healthcare professionals should reassure families that this phase is temporary and be given strategies to optimize success once the late preterm infant is medically stable, such as providing breast milk, building maternal breast milk supply, and breast nuzzling opportunities. This is the perfect time to show new parents the difference between nutritive and non-nutritive feedings.

Some infants will be able to effectively latch, suck, and swallow colostrum. Others will tire quickly, be unable to sustain nutritive sucking, or lack the strength to draw the nipple/areola into the mouth and generate the necessary pressure to secure the nipple in the mouth. Unless weight loss or jaundice is an issue, not every feed will need to be supplemented. Supplementation should only occur when the feed was not nutritive; i.e., no swallows occurred and the newborn had difficulty maintaining the latch, difficulty staying awake, and is vigorous at the breast for at least 15 min [5]. These are feeds that need supplementation. If the newborn is able to sustain a nutritive feed for at least 15 min, is vigorous throughout the feed, and had visible swallows, then not only is supplementation not necessary for that feed but also is limiting the infant's time at the breast [4]. For this feed, the newborn should be encouraged to stay at the breast as long as he is maintaining a nutritive feed. These nutritive and lively feeds will become more frequent as the newborn matures and is no longer affected by health challenges of prematurity such as hyper-bilirubinemia, unstable glucose levels, or infection. *Important to note that the road to effective feeding is not linear but vacillates day to day.*

8.5 · Supplementation: Evidence-Informed Strategies

Hospital discharge for the late preterm infant requires safe and successful feeding and a plan for optimal feeding [12–15]. Hospital supplementation will typically not exceed 20 ml post-breastfeed. As the newborn matures and their stomach grows, the supplementation amounts can be anywhere from 30–60 ml per feed depending on how well breastfeeding is going. Cup, spoon, and finger feeds are techniques typically used in hospital but are more difficult and time-consuming for families to perform at home. At home, the focus should be to have as many feeds at the breast as possible. A Supplemental Nutrition System (SNS) may help sustain a positive breastfeeding experience. The SNS consists of a small container that can be hung around the mother's neck filled with expressed breastmilk/formula. One or two tubes are connected to the container and secured to the mother's nipple. If using a nipple shield, the tube can be passed through one of the holes of the nipple shield prior to applying to the areola. Once the newborn latches onto both the areola and the SNS, he is able to obtain supplementation at the same time as feeding from the breast saving energy for the next feed. Once the necessary supplementation amount is achieved, the tube can be easily removed from the newborn's mouth and continue to feed at the breast until satiation or fatigue is achieved. This encourages the newborn to have as many feeds at the breast as possible and is the best solution for encouraging exclusive breastfeeding.

8.6   Bottle Feeding

Bottle feeding is a common supplemental mode for the late preterm infants. Infant suck-swallow-breathe skill, ability to communicate, position, parental skill, and bottle characteristics will all impact the late preterm infant's success with bottle feeding. In a recent study, it was observed that feeding difficulties in late preterm infants such as gagging, tongue thrusting, and choking existed regardless of whether the infant was fed at the breast or by bottle [1]. A review of bottle strategies will help ensure bottle feeding safety and success, whether used as a temporary measure toward breastfeeding or used as a sole feeding mode.

Bottle and nipple choice can impact whether a bottle feed is safe, effective, or pleasurable [16, 17]. During the postpartum stay, the late preterm infant may be introduced to a bottle and nipple provided by the hospital. Once feeding effectively, the newborn is deemed competent for discharge. However, once home, the late preterm infant will be exposed to a different bottle and nipple. If the experience of bottle feeding is no longer safe, effective, or pleasurable, feeding disorganization and stress result [8, 18]. Parents resort to purchasing a variety of bottles and nipples in desperate hope of finding a suitable bottle and nipple system for their baby. Commercial bottles and nipples vary in size, shape, flow rate, texture, and appearance. In the end, the late preterm infant is subjected to variable systems all while attempting to maintain physiologic stability and develop suck-swallow-breathe coordination.

- Nipple shape should be a regular shape. Late preterm infants often struggle to open their mouth widely to achieve a good latch and may only latch on the nub of a wide nipple. This shallow latch will contribute to poor transfer at the bottle, but perhaps, more importantly, this shallow latch may be transferred to breastfeeding and result in poor transfer and maternal discomfort. Avoidance of wide nipples is recommended until the late preterm infant is big enough to have a sufficient latch.

- Nipple choice should be a "slow flow" or "newborn" nipple [16, 19]: A significant difference in flow rate has been discovered among these nipples [10, 14, 16]. In addition, there is significant variability within the same nipple type [10, 16]. Parents may have to abandon one nipple manufacturer for another to find a nipple flow that their late preterm infant can safely feed from. Unfortunately, parents will not find useful information on manufacturer labels to guide purchase [10]. The "drip test" (tipping bottle down to observe drip rate) is not a valid test of a nipple; the baby's performance with a nipple is the best indicator of the appropriateness of the nipple.

- A simple strategy to facilitate transition home is to use the same supplies in hospital that the newborn will encounter at home. The healthcare professional can coach families to make evidence-informed choices if bottle feeding is necessary for the late preterm infant. Parents should be taught to look at their newborn's behavior and feeding quality when evaluating the success and safety of a bottle feed.

- Heat bottles without nipple attached to avoid building pressure in the bottle. Evidence of this pressure build-up may be seen as milk squirting out of the nipple when bottle is tipped horizontal. If bottles are heated with the nipple attached, parents can release the pressure by unscrewing the nipple and reattaching.

- As the volume in the bottle increases, so does the flow rate from the nipple [10]. For example, a 120 ml bottle containing 120 ml fluid will flow faster than a 120 ml bottle with 60 ml fluid. For the late preterm infant with flow coordination challenges, parents could experiment with less volume in a bottle to help reduce flow rate.

- The nipple ring should be snugly twisted onto the bottle but not overly tight. An overly tight connection between the nipple ring and bottle will result in a vacuum and make bottle feeding more challenging [20].

- Parents often misinterpret low bottle intake as a problem caused by the bottle flow rate and will introduce faster nipple flows. Faster nipples should be discouraged as the late preterm infant may not have sufficient suck-swallow-breathe coordination to safely consume milk from a faster nipple and choking may result. In addition, a faster flow rate from the bottle may lead to bottle preference and further complicate breastfeeding progress.

8.7   Newborn Bottle-Feeding Strategies

Bottle feeding strategies to avoid:

- Twisting, jiggling, or moving the bottle nipple in the baby's mouth while the baby is taking a breathing and/or swallowing break or has fallen asleep.
- Letting baby suck too fast without breathing or taking rest breaks.
- Persistent coaxing or forced feeds despite infant cues of satiation or exhaustion.

These strategies are not recommended as the infant will learn that feeding is not pleasurable [14]. In addition, these noxious experiences will interrupt the newborn's need to rest and breathe [20].

Until satiation cues are clear, it may be easy for late preterm infants to overconsume during bottle feeds as the milk drips by gravity into their mouth from the bottle, or parents may overly coax newborns to finish the bottle. Overconsumption can contribute to gastrointestinal upset and gastroesophageal reflux. Overconsumption will also interfere with breastfeeding.

Optimal feeding strategies include the following:

- A side-lying elevated position for bottle feeding may facilitate feeding success for the late preterm infant. This position is similar to the breastfeeding position with the ear and shoulder up and the sternum and face in alignment. The parent should be able to clearly see the newborn's face to monitor the feeding effectively. This position allows greater control of the bottle flow, reduced gravitational dripping into newborn's mouth, and enhanced newborn postural stability and comfort [20]. Parents should be reassured that this is a temporary measure and a semi-upright position may be introduced once feeding consistency is established.

- A short rest break, of up to one minute, during bottle feeding can be an effective strategy to help preterm newborns maintain respiratory reserves and enhance feeding endurance [20].

- Encourage parents to watch for cues of satiation; however, recognize that late preterm infants may not clearly communicate cues of satiation yet. Until satiation is consistently communicated, parent can use other signs to indicate adequate intake, such as number of wet diapers, stooling pattern, sleep duration, and weight gain pattern.

- During bottle feeding, parents should monitor for suck-swallow-breathe incoordination as evidenced by spillage, restlessness, anxious facial expressions, long suck bursts without pauses, arching, coughing, or choking. Newborns are innately programmed to suck fast and hard at the beginning of feeds to establish letdown from the breast. This behavior on a bottle often results in rapid milk transfer, gulping, long sucking pattern without breathing, and rapid stomach filling. Until infants demonstrate a slower suck rate, parents can slow the feed down by "pacing" or intermittently interrupting the rapid sucking pattern [7, 14]. The nipple may be tipped to stop the flow of milk, but this may result in sucking air and gassiness. Ideally, the nipple should be removed entirely from the mouth and left resting on the infant's lip [20]. The feed continues as soon as the infant has swallowed, taken a couple breaths and cued desire to resume feeding. Parents may need to do this every 3–8 sucks until the sucking rate slows down. Eventually the newborn will demonstrate self-pacing as evidenced by brief pauses, suck-swallow-breathe coordination, and a relaxed, enjoyable feeding.

Bottle feeding is a reality for many late preterm infants. Ideally the bottle supplement is a temporary measure as breastfeeding improves. In the meantime, parents can make the bottle feed as safe and pleasurable as possible. As the late preterm infant matures, suck strength, stamina, and suck-swallow-breathe coordination will improve, and the feeding experience will change. Parents should understand the signs of suck-swallow-breathe incoordination and strategies to intervene. With consistent strategies, the infant learns to trust the feed experience and to feed more effectively and efficiently.

8.8   Weaning Off Supplementation

A variety of weaning tips to facilitate exclusive breastfeeding are available for families, but few are research-based for the late preterm infant population. Again, the evidence from the general preterm population and very preterm population and expert opinion are applied to the late preterm infant. Two contrasting case studies will be used to illustrate use of the strategies cited in this chapter.

8.8.1   Case # 1

Adele, born at 35 weeks, with good breastfeeding skill is developing milk transfer skills. Mother reports swallowing at the breast. Adele needs small "top ups" of breast milk after breastfeeds. Adele's mother is alternating breast and supplemental feeds.

8.8.2   Case # 2

Mohammed, born at 36 weeks, with early breastfeeding skill has a heavy reliance on supplemental feeds. Sometimes he is too fussy to latch and sometimes he nuzzles on the breast for long periods but transfers very little. His hunger cues are subtle and not consistent. Mohammed's mother is offering breastfeeding twice a day.

8.8.3   Encouraging more Frequent Breastfeeding

For these two newborns, we will apply a strategy to encourage more frequent breastfeeding.

> Simply put, practice makes perfect. Offering the breast once a day will not promote breastfeeding. Multiple short breastfeeding practice sessions along with supplementary feeds will facilitate breastfeeding skill. Inform the family that there will be feeding quality inconsistencies from feed to feed and day to day [12]. The healthcare professional can individualize a discharge feeding plan with breastfeeding frequency and duration recommendations.

For Adele, the feeding plan could recommend breastfeeding at each feed for up to 20–25 min and offering a supplemental feed for 5–10 min. Adele may need a short rest after breastfeeding or a diaper change to help her arouse for supplemental feeding. Parents are cautioned to avoid long feeding duration. Alternatively, Adele's supplemental method could include a small volume by tube or syringe during breastfeeding, thus eliminating the need to interrupt breastfeeding for supplementation.

Mohammed's feeding plan may recommend breastfeeding at each feed for several minutes or longer, depending on his behavior at the breast. Mohammed's family should be aware of signs of milk transfer at the breast. As breastfeeding skill and interest improve, breastfeeding duration may increase. Supplemental feeds will initially be close to a total feed and will decrease overtime. Family should be aware of signs of hunger and satiation and be taught to provide supplemental volumes accordingly.

Weaning supplementation is another strategy we'll apply to these two cases: wean supplemental volumes gradually over time. Families often struggle to know how much and when to give a supplemental feed [3]. Once the late preterm infant is breastfeeding with good signs of milk transfer, the family may gradually initiate weaning:

(a) Periodic weight to monitor progress, e. g., bimonthly, weekly, or biweekly as needed [3, 12]. Primary care provider will track weight gain and growth patterns [5].
(b) Use semi-demand feeding routine until hunger cues are consistent [21]. Help infant arouse every 2–4 h, depending on the quality of the preceding feed [3].
(c) Determine need for supplement by monitoring adequacy of breast milk intake: weight gain pattern, satiation after feeds, sleep patterns, and stooling and voiding patterns [22].
(d) An intake diary may help families denote feeding patterns, e.g., see overall impact of breastfeeding duration or quality of feed, long feeding duration, large or small supplemental feeds, and change over time.
(e) Gradually wean supplemental volumes and compare infant behavior and satiation.
(f) Following "good" breastfeeding sessions, experiment with no supplement, and compare infant behavior.

Adele's breastfeeding progressed well over time, and the family noted she was more and more satiated after 20–25 min breastfeeds. They discovered that she was less and less interested in the "top up" supplement after breastfeeding. Adele would arouse consistently every 2–3 h with hunger signs and was gaining weight sufficiently. The family eventually discontinued supplementation.

Mohammed's breastfeeding sessions were showing signs of improvement as he is now latching for 5–20 min for every breast feed. Sometimes he only needed a half-volume "top up," and sometimes he required full supplementation. The variable volumes indicate inconsistent milk transfer and family attentiveness to his feeding cues, i.e., not forcing the same volume after every breastfeed. Weight gain has been low, and Mohammed's mother is discouraged. Mohammed's family requires continued support by healthcare professionals for breastfeeding, for weight gain promotion, and eventually for weaning strategies. Weekly weights and lactation support are arranged at the public health office.

8.9   Managing Parents Expectations with Education

Ideally, the late preterm infant should be seen by a healthcare provider 1–2 days after discharge and as often as necessary thereafter to ensure adequate weight gain. Once a pattern of weight gain has been established, anticipatory guidance should be offered to transition to a more demand-type feeding regimen, especially at night, to ease the burden on the family of maintaining a more rigid, time-controlled feeding schedule. The clinician should work with the family to develop a strategy that permits as much direct feeding at breast as possible. The two primary goals are ensuring that maternal milk supply is protected and that the infant receives sufficient hydration and nutrition. Often, "triple feeding" is recommended, which involves attempting to feed at the breast followed by use of a breast pump and feeding any expressed milk to infant. This plan can sometimes be difficult to sustain as it involves a lot of planning and routines. It is important that the healthcare provider be a source of support throughout this plan.

Although new mothers will want to discontinue routine pumping as soon as possible, it is important to remind them that the pump is doing the work of maintaining the milk supply because their late preterm infant does not have the ability of doing so at the moment. As the infant matures, they will progressively consume more milk at the breast and require less supplemented volume. Mothers are encouraged to maintain pumping in the meantime, often with six sessions during the day and one at night (between the hours of midnight—five when the prolactin levels are the highest). Do not routinely offer a bottle after each feeding; do not routinely pump after each feeding.

When families of late preterm infants are not informed about prematurity or are misled to believe that their newborns are simply small full-term newborns, they are not prepared for the challenges and time required to facilitate good weight gain, effective feeding, and progress toward exclusive breastfeeding. The workload of breastfeeds, supplementary feeds, and pumping can be overwhelming. The patience and diligence required for each feed can be exasperating. Families may abandon preconceived breastfeeding goals. Healthcare providers can improve late preterm infant breastfeeding rates by helping families set realistic expectations in hospital, being prepared with multiple strategies, and building supportive professional- and community-based support networks. When meeting with parents of late preterm infants post-discharge, one of the most common themes that arises is their dissatisfaction and disappointment in their breastfeeding experience. They will discuss their sadness that they had to give their newborn formula, that the length of time dedicated to feeding is exhausting and not what they expected, that there are difficulties and challenges with breast pumping, and that they feel an overall grieving of their idealized breastfeeding journey. Parents need to be told that most late preterm infants will not feed effectively immediately after birth and that it is normal. Parents need to also be informed that those early feeding interactions will set the stage for feeding behaviors to come in both infants and mothers. Interest in feeding and length of time the infant can sustain a latch and mature their suck-swallow skills may vary at feedings. An awareness of the unique characteristics of late preterm infants will help families be realistic in their feeding experience after hospital discharge.

Families should not assume the late preterm infant is yet able to consume sufficient intake from the breast and must monitor for other signs of satiation, such as weight gain, relaxed muscle tone, wet diapers, stooling pattern, and sleep duration. For late preterm infants with lingering low milk transfer at the breast, or medical issues such as hyperbilirubinemia or hypoglycemia, supplemental feeds are a necessity [3, 23, 24]. Families need guidance to develop a realistic feeding plan and community-based supports to wean from supplementation [22].

Counsel parents that exclusive breastfeeding will take at least a month following hospital discharge [24]. During this time, infants benefit from multiple practice opportunities to build breastfeeding skills and reflexes. Mothers also need to build and protect an adequate breast milk supply so that the milk is freely available as their newborn learns to breastfeed [25]. Once maternal supply and infant breastfeeding skill are in progress, a weaning plan may be introduced.

Families, and in particular, mothers of late preterm infants will need family or community support. The maternal workload "triple threat" (breastfeeding, supplemental feeding, and pumping) is time- and energy-consuming [21]. Lack of family support contributes to shorter breastfeeding duration [26]. Mothers are encouraged to seek help early on from community services, breastfeeding support groups, and even lactation consultants when necessary. Parental stress related to feeding has been recognized in this population [3] and can interfere with parent-infant bonding [27]. Exhaustion, anxiety, worry, isolation, and lack of support are identified by mothers of premature newborns [26, 28]. The benefits of family support can be seen in our two case studies:

- Adele's family managed well with feedings at home with limited support from health-care professionals. Extended family provided good support and help in the home.
- Mohammed's family was well supported by extended family. Mohammed's mother was able to balance baby's care and pumping time. Family members helped promote maternal rest and nutrition. Mohammed's mother required ongoing lactation support to optimize milk transfer during breastfeeding, such as deepening his latch, and maternal breast massage and compression. Ongoing reinforcement of cue-based feeding and periodic weights continued while Mohammed learned to breastfeed more effectively.

Healthcare professionals should encourage mothers to activate support networks to help with activities of daily living such as rest, nutrition, fluid intake, household activities, and caring for older children [28]. Lactation support should be offered to mothers with inadequate milk supply or breastfeeding challenges [23, 25, 29]. Ideally, health professional support and support groups in the community should be identified predischarge to provide seamless transition for the families with late preterm infants [3, 21, 25, 30]. Effective post-discharge follow-up for vulnerable preterm infants is associated with decreased need for emergency department visits or readmission [18].

Conclusion

Late preterm infants are not easy to feed at first. Guidance is required for parents to navigate their feeding journey. Parents need to understand that feeding skills take time to develop as well they need to understand how they may help their newborn. Patience, consistent strategies, and practice are key. Exclusive breast-feeding goals can be reached with a realistic perspective, a variety of strategies, and strong community supports. Parents should be informed as to when and how to seek healthcare professional advice if feedings are stressful. Healthcare professionals can assist parents to become confident with feeding their infant and foster safe, pleasurable feedings for both infant and parent [8].

References

1. Premji S, Currie G, Reilly S, Dosani A, Oliver LM, Lodha AK, Young M. A qualitative study: mothers of late preterm infants relate their experiences of community-based care. PLoS One. 2017;12(3):e0174419. https://doi.org/10.1371/journal.pone.0174419.
2. DeMauro SB, Patel PR, Medoff-Cooper B, Posencheg M, Abbasi S. Postdischarge feeding patterns in early- and late-preterm infants. Clin Pediatr. 2011;50(10):957–62. https://doi.org/10.1177/0009922811409028.
3. Dosani AH, Hemraj J, Premji SS, Currie G, Reilly SM, Lodha AK, et al. Breastfeeding the late preterm infant: experiences of mothers and perceptions of public health nurses. Int Breastfeed J. 2017;12:23. https://doi.org/10.1186/s13006-017-0114-0.
4. Ludwig SM. Oral feeding and the late preterm infant. Newborn Infant Nurs Rev. 2007;7(2):72–5. https://doi.org/10.1053/j.nainr.2007.05.005.
5. Meier P, Wright K, Engstrom J. Management of breastfeeding during and after the maternity hospitalization for late preterm infants. Clin Perinatol. 2013;40(4):689–705. https://doi.org/10.1016/j.clp.2013.07.014.
6. Mattson E, Funkquist EL, Wickström M, Nqvist KH, Volgsten H. Healthy late preterm infants and supplementary artificial milk feeds: effects on breast feeding and associated parameters. Midwifery. 2015;31(4):426–31. https://doi.org/10.1016/j.midw.2014.12.004.
7. White A, Parnell K. The transition from tube to full oral feeding (breast or bottle) – a cue-based developmental approach. J Neonatal Nurs. 2013;19(4):189–97. https://doi.org/10.1016/j.jnn.2013.03.006.
8. Browne JV, Ross ES. Eating as a neurodevelopmental process for high-risk newborns. Clin Perinatol. 2011;38(4):731–43. https://doi.org/10.1016/j.clp.2011.08.004.
9. Walker M. Breastfeeding management for the late preterm infant: practical Interventions for "little imposters". Clin Lactat. 2010;1(1):22–6. https://doi.org/10.1891/215805310807011873.
10. Brackett, K. B. Know the flow, don't go with the flow! By Britt Pados PhD(c), RN, NNP-BC, bpados@email.unc.edu. Pediatric Feeding News; 2014. Available from http://pediatricfeedingnews.com/know-the-flow-dont-go-with-the-flow-by-britt-pados-phdc-rn-nnp-bc-bpadose-mail-unc-edu/. Accessed 28 Mar 2018.
11. Walker M. Breastfeeding the late preterm infant. J Obstet Gynecol Neonatal Nurs. 2008;37(6):692–701. https://doi.org/10.1111/j.1552-6909.2008.00293.x.
12. Gianni ML, Roggero P, Piemontese P, Liotto N, Orsi A, Amato OR, et al. Is nutritional support needed in late preterm infants? BMC Pediatr. 2015;15:194. https://doi.org/10.1186/s12887-015-0511-8.
13. Jefferies AL, Canadian Paediatric Society, Fetus and Newborn Committee. Going home: facilitating discharge of the preterm infant. Paediatric Child Health. 2014;19(1):31–42.

14. Sables-Baus S, DeSanto K, Henderson S, Kunz JL, Morris AC, Shields L, et al. Infant-directed oral feeding for premature and critically ill hospitalized infants: Guideline for practice. Chicago, IL: National Association of Neonatal Nurses; 2013.
15. Whyte RK, Canadian Paediatric Society, Fetus and Newborn Committee. Safe discharge of the late preterm infant: position statement. Paediatric Child Health. 2010;15(10):655–60.
16. Jackman KT. Go with the flow: choosing a feeding system for infants in the neonatal intensive care unit and beyond based on flow performance. Newborn Infant Nurs Rev. 2013;13(1):31–4.
17. Raines D. Preparing for NICU discharge: mothers' concerns. Neonatal Netw. 2013;32(6):399–403. https://doi.org/10.1891/0730-0832.32.6.399.
18. Vonderheid SC, Rankin K, Norr K, Vasa R, Hills S, White-Trau R. Health care use outcomes of an integrated hospital-to-home mother-preterm infant intervention. J Obstet Gynecol Neonatal Nurs. 2016;45(5):625–38. https://doi.org/10.1016/j.jogn.2016.05.007.
19. Lau C, Sheena HR, Shulman RJ, Schanler RJ. Oral feeding in low birth weight infants. J Pediatr. 1997;130(4):561–9.
20. Shaker CS. Infant-guided, co-regulated feeding in the neonatal intensive care unit. Part II: interventions to promote neuroprotection and safety. Semin Speech Lang. 2017;38(2):106–15. https://doi.org/10.1055/s-0037-1599108.
21. Lucas R, Paquett R, Briere CE, McGrath JG. Furthering our understanding of the needs of mothers who are pumping breast milk for infants in the NICU: an integrative review. Adv Neonatal Care. 2014;14(4):214–52. https://doi.org/10.1097/ANC.0000000000000110.
22. Cleaveland K. Feeding challenges in the late preterm infant. Neonatal Netw. 2010;29(1):37–41. https://doi.org/10.1891/0730-0832.29.37.
23. Hubbard ET, Stellwagen L, Wolf A. The late preterm infant: a little baby with big needs. Contemp Pediatr. 2007;24(11):51–8.
24. Meier PF, Furman LM, Degenhardt M. Increased lactation risk for late preterm infants and mothers: evidence and management strategies to protect breastfeeding. J Midwifery Womens Health. 2007;52(6):579–87.
25. Briere CE, McGrath J, Cong X, Cusson R. An integrative review of factors that influence breastfeeding duration for premature infants after NICU hospitalization. J Obstet Gynecol Neonatal Nurs. 2014;43(3):272–81. https://doi.org/10.1111/1552-6909.12297.
26. Phillips-Pula L, Pickler R, McGrath JM, Brown LF, Dusing SC. Caring for a preterm infant at home: a mother's perspective. J Perinat Neonat Nurs. 2013;27(4):335–44. https://doi.org/10.1097/JPN.0b013e3182a983be.
27. Silberstein D, Feldman R, Gardner JM, Karmel BZ, Kuint J, Geva R. The mother-infant feeding relationship across the first year and the development of feeding difficulties in low-risk premature infants. Infancy. 2009;14(5):501–25.
28. Purdy IB, Singh N, Le C, Bell C, Whiteside C, Collins M. Biophysiologic and social stress relationships with breast milk feeding pre- and post-discharge from the neonatal intensive care unit. J Obstet Gynecol Neonatal Nurs. 2012;41(3):347–57. https://doi.org/10.1111/j.1552-6909.2012.01368.x.
29. Munson M, Saatkamp R, West C. Late preterm infants: steps to success. Neonatal Netw. 2011;30(4):267–70. https://doi.org/10.1891/0730-0832.30.4.267.
30. Lee SY, Guan JJ. Prevalence and prediators of exclusive breastfeeding in late preterm infants at 12 weeks. Child Health Nurs Res. 2016;22(2):79–86. https://doi.org/10.4094/chnr.2016.22.2.79.

Late Preterm Infants and Neurodevelopmental Outcomes: Why Do I Need to Serve and Return?

Aliyah Dosani, Dianne Creighton, and Abhay K. Lodha

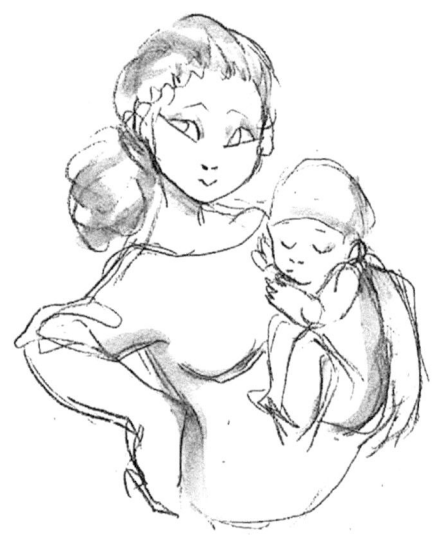

A. Dosani (✉)
School of Nursing and Midwifery, Mount Royal University, Calgary, AB, Canada
e-mail: adosani@mtroyal.ca

Department of Community Health Sciences, Cumming School of Medicine, University of Calgary, Calgary, AB, Canada

D. Creighton
Neonatal Follow-Up Clinic, Alberta Children's Hospital, Calgary, AB, Canada

Department of Paediatrics, Cumming School of Medicine, University of Calgary, Calgary, AB, Canada
e-mail: dianne.creighton@ahs.ca

A. K. Lodha
Department of Paediatrics, Cumming School of Medicine, University of Calgary, Calgary, AB, Canada

Department of Community Health Sciences, Cumming School of Medicine, University of Calgary, Calgary, AB, Canada

Department of Paeditrics, Foothills Medical Center C211, Alberta Health Services, Calgary, AB, Canada
e-mail: aklodha@ucalgary.ca

© Springer International Publishing AG, part of Springer Nature 2019
S. S. Premji (ed.), *Late Preterm Infants*, https://doi.org/10.1007/978-3-319-94352-7_9

9.1   Background

The survival rate of late preterm infants (LPIs) is as high as 99% [1]. At the population level, morbidity and mortality rates of LPIs are higher than term infants, and the outcomes of LPIs are not the same as infants who are born at term [2–6]. The common immediate morbidities experienced by LPIs such as feeding difficulties [7–9], trouble regulating temperature (hypothermia) [10, 11], low blood sugar [12], respiratory morbidities (especially transient tachypnea of the newborns and hypoxic lung injury) [13], and jaundice [14, 15] have additional impacts on long-term neurodevelopment (ND).

The long-term ND outcomes of LPIs are not well studied and described. This chapter will therefore describe the long-term impact of being born LPI due to incomplete brain development. ND outcomes at various ages including 0–12 months, 18–24 months, 36 months, and 5 years are presented based on available research. The existing information reflects significant underestimation of the magnitude of the issue. To conclude, we will consider various interventions that may be effective in preventing the severity of the neurodevelopmental impairments (NDI). We will show that LPI birth has substantial public health consequences and burden on society, including the educational system.

9.2   Brain Development

When compared to infants born at full term, LPIs have a smaller brain size and less developed components of the brain (e.g., myelination of the posterior limb of the internal capsule and immature gyral folding). These changes could be connected to the ND problems in LPIs [16, 17]. The last half of pregnancy is vital for the brain to grow; the brain continues to develop and mature beyond birth [18]. From 34 weeks to term, 65% of the brain is developed, but there are critical components (the gray matter, the white matter, and the cerebral cortex) that have not been fully developed [18, 19]. During this developing phase, the change from intrauterine to extrauterine alters the way in which the brain develops and has long-term consequences on neurodevelopment [16, 18]. Figure 9.1 identifies potential contributing factors that may adversely impact neurodevelopment. Neonatal factors including infection, low blood sugar (hypoglycemia), a high level of jaundice, hemorrhage in the brain (intraventricular hemorrhage), difficulty breathing (resulting in hypoxic respiratory failure) and lack of oxygen to the brain (hypoxic ischemic injury), and other maternal factors, like intra-amniotic infection (chorioamnionitis), may have additional impacts on brain development and outcomes [20].

There is a critical period in development where various structures and pathways in the brain are formed [21]. Total brain volume increases in a steady linear fashion [18], and, during the last 10 weeks of gestation, the gray matter increases fourfold [22]. It is the early electrical activity that takes place in the brain (specifically the neuronal networks) during this time that is essential to brain development [23]. In addition, the early neonatal period involves a marked increase in total physical

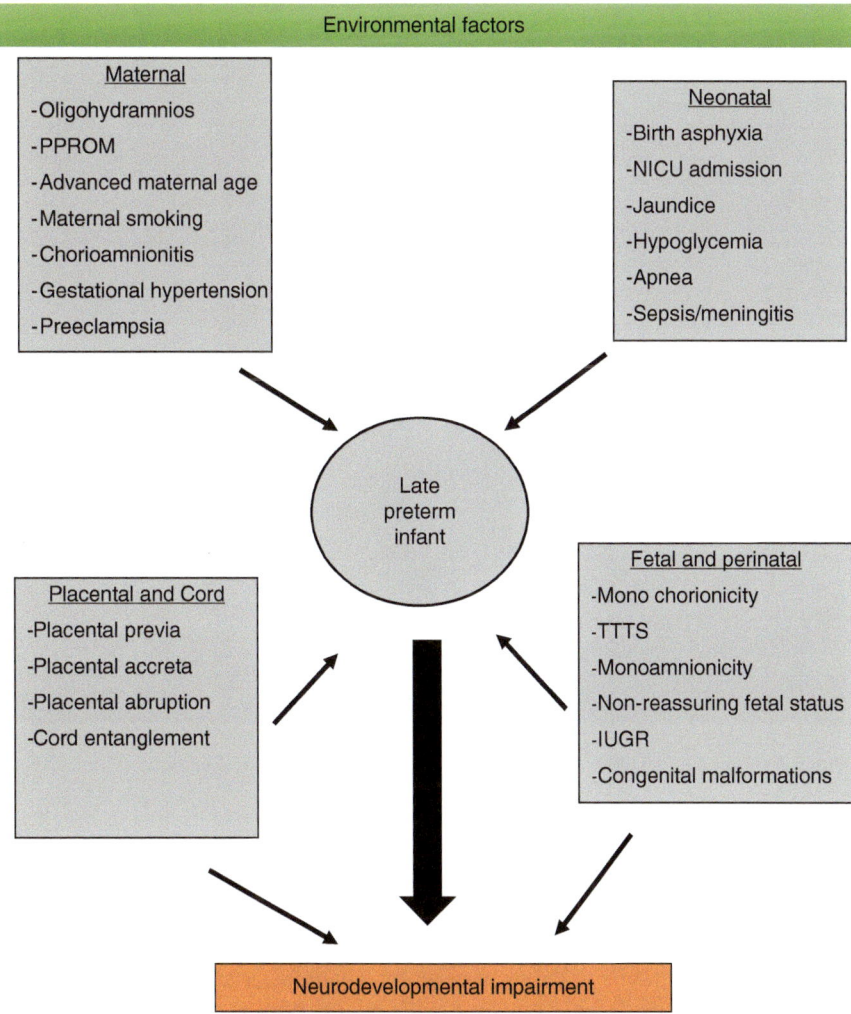

Fig. 9.1 Potential factors contributing to neurodevelopmental impairment. *PPROM* preterm premature rupture of membranes; *NICU* neonatal intensive care unit; *TITS* twin-twin transfusion syndrome; *IUGR* intrauterine growth restriction

connections and interactions between neurons in the cerebral cortex, demonstrating a relationship between early brain activity and brain growth [23, 24]. The white matter in LPIs is still developing and is more at risk for injury that may result in long-term effects compared to the term infant population [25]. See Appendix 1 for brain development in LPIs that occurs in the last half of gestation and Fig. 9.2 for the process of brain maturation in a preterm infant. As depicted in the figure, maturation improves over time as demonstrated in the increase in the folded appearance of the brain. As a result, any insult or injury may have impact on long-term outcome.

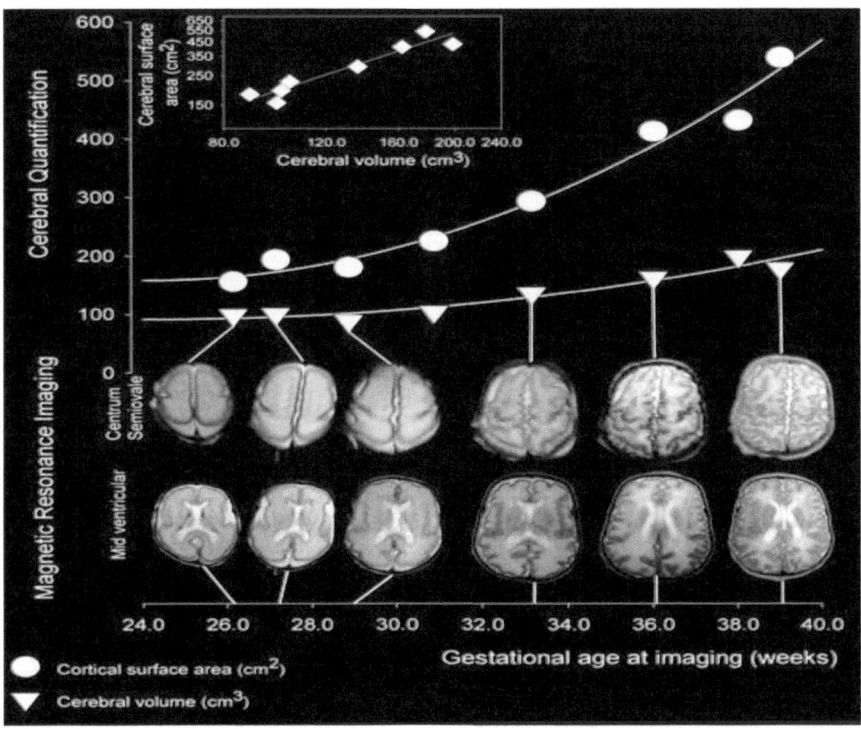

Fig. 9.2 Maturation of the brain in normal female preterm infant [26] (Reproduced from Kapellou et al. [90])

9.3   Neurodevelopmental Impairments/Outcomes

The NDIs of healthy LPIs when compared to healthy term infants are different. LPI birth may result in NDI in the form of motor, cognitive, academic, behavioral, and psychological issues when compared with infants born at term [20, 25, 27, 28]. These impairments may be related to alterations in brain growth and development of LPIs [29].

9.3.1   0–12 Months

Jaundice (hyperbilirubinemia) is the most significant morbidity that can occur in the early neonatal period that could cause long-term damage (known as kernicterus) to the LPI newborn brain. Specifically, it is the free unconjugated bilirubin that causes brain damage [30]. It is important to note that the precise level at which hyperbilirubinemia becomes toxic is unknown [30], mainly because the total serum/plasma bilirubin level is not the most precise indicator of brain damage (neurotoxicity) [31]. However, LPIs are at a higher risk of developing kernicterus than term infants and demonstrate clinical manifestations of brain damage from jaundice (known as bilirubin neurotoxicity) at an earlier postnatal age than term infants possibly due to weak blood brain barrier [32]. The clinical manifestations of kernicterus can be divided into three main types: initial phase, intermediate phase, and advanced phase. During the initial phase, the infant is observed to exhibit a slight stupor (lethargic and sleepy) and demonstrate little movement with slight hypotonia, poor sucking, and a slightly high-pitched cry [33]. In the intermediate phase, the infant demonstrates moderate stupor, irritability, variable tone (usually increased, some with abnormal posturing termed retrocollis-opisthotonos), minimal feeding, and a high-pitched cry [33]. The advanced phase is characterized by the infant exhibiting deep stupor to coma, has increased tone with pronounced posturing, not feeding, and a shrill cry [33].

With respect to their neurodevelopmental profile, infants born at 34 weeks of gestational age (GA) are different than infants born at 35 and 36 weeks of GA in their tone, Moro reflex, and visual orientation [34]. When assessed at term age, LPIs born at 34 weeks of GA resembled the neurologic profile of very preterm infants who were assessed at term equivalent age, with less flexor tone in the limbs (including both traction and recoil), lower head control, a higher rate of brisk reflexes, and stronger palmar grasps, startles, and tremors [34, 35]. LPIs have a higher risk of developmental delay between 34 and 41 weeks of life [36]. With respect to motor development, when compared to term infants, LPIs at 6, 9, and 12 months corrected gestational age (CGA) have been demonstrated to have lower tone and reflexes [37]. The observed difference in neurologic profile between infants born at 34 weeks of GA and infants born at 35 and 36 weeks of GA can be attributed to the critical period of brain growth and development in terms of the increasing volume of both gray and myelinated white matter as mentioned above. However, motor assessments of LPIs in the first year of life do not predict their ND outcome at 4 years of age [38]. Therefore, it is important to conduct follow-up assessments at 3, 9, 18–24 months and at 4 years of age [38].

9.3.2   18–24 Months

Late preterm infants have developmental outcomes that are worse than term infants at 24 months of age [39]. In addition, LPIs have double the risk for adverse ND outcomes at 24 months of age, with majority of deficiencies identified in the cognitive domain [40]. At 24 months of CGA, LPIs have delayed language and motor development when compared with infants born at term, with the disparity being the greatest in language development [29, 41, 42]. Compared with term infants, LPIs have increased odds of experiencing more severe cognitive delay, milder cognitive developmental delay, severe psychomotor developmental delay, and milder psychomotor developmental delay at 24 months of CGA [39]. Furthermore, LPIs demonstrate poorer social competence [29] at 24 months CGA. Interestingly, LPIs who have larger total brain tissue, white matter, and cerebellar volumes at term equivalent age demonstrate better ND outcomes at 24 months of CGA [43]. These poorer

NDI may be due to LPIs experiencing widespread white matter microstructural alterations compared with term equivalent age [25]. This suggests that brain volumes may be a significant marker for neurodevelopment in LPIs [43]. While alterations in brain growth and development could be related to the NDI observed, various risk factors have also been identified. These risk factors include male sex, socioeconomic disadvantage, nonwhite ethnic origin, preeclampsia, and not receiving breast milk at discharge [40].

9.3.3   36 Months

The language, speech, and executive functions are not well developed before 24 months. Large studies from Norway and the USA found that LPIs were at increased risk of communication and expressive language impairments at age 18 and 36 months [44, 45]. However, based on historical cohort studies and small unpowered prospective studies, the ND outcome at 18–24 months of CGA is not predictive of future long-term ND outcomes. Due to limited resources and financial constraints, follow-up in the form of multidisciplinary clinics for LPIs is not well-established. Furthermore, LPIs comprise up to 75% of the preterm population, making their follow-up difficult, based on sheer volume alone.

9.3.4   36 Months: School Age

LPIs admitted to NICU and those of male sex are at a greater risk of cognitive deficit in early childhood, specifically poor general conceptual ability, nonverbal reasoning, and visual-spatial scores than term-born children [46–49]. These NDIs may be due to late maturation of the brain (specifically, frontal-cortical and frontal-subcortical regions), lack of oxygen or blood supply (i.e., hypoxic or ischemic events), and/or infection or inflammation in parts of the brain (specifically white matter) [46]. Longitudinal studies with large sample sizes from various countries around the world demonstrate LPIs have a higher incidence of cerebral palsy; mental retardation; disorders of psychological development, behavior, and emotion; other major disabilities including blindness, poor vision, hearing loss, and seizure disorders; and medical disability severely affecting working capacity [50–52]. LPIs have an increased risk of cerebral palsy if they have had resuscitation at birth, antibiotic treatment during the first hospitalization, 1-min Apgar score < 7, and intracranial hemorrhage [52].

Large studies have found that LPI births are associated with an increased risk of poorer educational achievement at age 5 years, possibly a result of a smaller and less mature brain at the time of birth [53–55]. LPIs are also at risk of suspension in kindergarten at 3 and 4 years of age [36]. There is inconclusive evidence in the literature with respect to school readiness, reading, and math scores of LPIs. Part of the issue lies in the use of various measurement tools. Woythaler and colleagues [39] found that LPIs between the ages of 5 and 6 years have lower scores for total school readiness, reading, math, and expressive language. Chyi and colleagues [56] present similar results. However, the reading skills may resolve by the third and fifth grade [57]. Poorer language performance may be identified as early as 20 months and continue until 8 years of age [42].

In grade 3, LPIs have lower scores for math and English compared to term infants [58]. Interestingly, there is a linear association between gestational age at birth and test scores until 39 weeks of gestation. Teachers of LPIs in grade 5 have some concerns about their learning abilities, and they sometimes require intervention in the form of special education [56, 58]. Interestingly, a dose-dependent relationship also exists with LPI gestational age at birth and special educational needs [59].

LPIs are at the risk for socioemotional problems at 6 years of age demonstrated by IQ scores below 85 [51]. Furthermore, LPIs experience attention, behavioral, and internalizing behavior disorders in the later grades and externalizing aggressive behavior disorder in later grades, and this may manifest as having difficulties in school [36, 47, 49, 56, 57, 60, 61]. In large cohort studies, a higher number of LPIs were prescribed attention deficit hyperactivity disorder (ADHD) medication between 6 and 19 years [62, 63]. However, conflicting evidence exists in the literature which indicates that former late preterm infants have similar rates of learning disabilities and ADHD as term infants [64]. By age 7, LPIs may exhibit motor coordination difficulties [65].

9.4   Multidisciplinary Neurodevelopmental Assessments

In Table 9.1, proposed timing of assessment by age conducted by various health-care professionals is presented. It is especially important that in-depth assessments are done in a timely way to identify possible ND problem(s). This will facilitate the implementation

Table 9.1 Proposed timing of assessment by age

Age	Assessments
4 months	Nursing and physician assessment, general physical examination, neurological examination, physiotherapy assessment, ophthalmology examination, social work assessment, and audiology screening
8 months	Nursing and physician assessment, general physical examination, neurological examination, audiology screening and nutrition
18–21 months	Nursing review, physiotherapy, psychology, speech/language pathology, and social work
36 months	Nursing review, general physical and neurological examination, psychology, speech/language pathology, orthoptics (eye care profession whose primary emphasis is the diagnosis and nonsurgical management of wandering eye, lazy eye and eye movement disorders), and social work
5 years	Nursing review, general physical and neurological examination, psychology, speech/language pathology, and social work. This visit may be offered to only children at greater risk of difficulties which become evident only near school age or who have behavioral problems

Table 9.2 Definitions of NDI

Impairments	Any NDI (any one or more of the following)	Significant or severe NDI (any one or more of the following)
Motor	Cerebral palsy with GMFCS I or higher, Bayley-III motor composite <85	Cerebral palsy with GMFCS III, IV, or V, Bayley-III motor composite <70
Cognitive	Bayley-III cognitive composite <85	Bayley-III cognitive composite <70
Language	Bayley-III language composite <70	Bayley-III language composite <70
Hearing	Sensorineural/mixed hearing loss	Hearing aid or cochlear implant
Vision	Unilateral or bilateral visual impairment	Bilateral visual impairment

GMFCS gross motor function classification system

of early intervention to promote brain development in LPIs. The timing of visits to various health-care professionals for appropriate assessments is tailored by availability of resources, nature of high-risk population, the type of surveillance used, and the purpose of the visits. Frequency of visits is usually linked to key developmental milestones.

9.5 Definitions of Neurodevelopmental Impairment in Preterm Infants

Once a potential issue with NDI has been identified, it is important for health-care providers to identify the scope of the issue. NDI has been classified into two groups based on severity of impairment: Any NDI and significant or severe NDI (Table 9.2) [66]. Please refer to Appendix 2 for an in-depth discussion of the NDI identification methods listed in Table 9.2. Common developmental tests for cognitive, language, and speech assessments at various ages are presented in Appendix 3.

9.5.1 Cerebral Palsy

Severity of motor dysfunction in cerebral palsy is classified into two categories: mild or moderate-severe. Mild cerebral palsy is defined as having abnormal tone and reflexes with no limiting effects on daily activities and functions. Moderate-severe cerebral palsy is defined as motor dysfunction requiring appliances or assistance with performance of daily activities and functions [67]. GMFCS (Gross Motor Function Classification System) is used to classify the severity of functional impairment in children with cerebral palsy [68]. In the absence of GMFCS information, cerebral palsy also refers to a nonprogressive disability of movement and posture and is diagnosed on the basis of abnormal muscle tone and reflexes on the physical and neurological examination.

9.5.2 Abnormal Language

Delays in language development are more common than delays in any other infant and child developmental domain [69]. Language is the most difficult to assess or observe because infants generally do not vocalize words spontaneously in front of health-care professionals. Between 10 and 18 months, it is helpful to keep track of the number of words the child expresses [69]. After 18 months this becomes more difficult as language usually increases exponentially [69]. Therefore, it is necessary for parents to be aware of their infant and young child reaching various language developmental milestones, as presented in Table 9.3. Receptive skills refer to the ability of the infant to understand language [69]. Expressive skills refer to the ability of the infant to make their thoughts, ideas, and expression known to others, in the form of speech, gestures, sign language, and body language [69]. It is important for parents to understand that the terms language and speech are not used interchangeably. A child can demonstrate normal language progression but be unable to speak as speech is one form of language [69]. Overall abnormal

Table 9.3 Language development milestones [69]

Periods of language development	Age	Characteristics
Pre-speech period	0–10 months	*Receptive language*: Ability to localize sounds like a bell; at 5 months can assume a posture that indicates the infant is "listening" and may engage in "vocal tennis" with the speaker. *Expressive language*: Ability to make vowel-like sounds; at 3 months the infant can vocalize after an adult has spoken; at 6 months the infant adds consonants to the vowels and "babbles"
Naming period	10–18 months	The infant realizes that people have names and objects have labels The infant begins to use words appropriately after they have been enforced (e.g., mama) Infants begin to recognize their own names and understand the meaning of the word "no" By 12 months infants can understand up to 100 words and can follow a command if the speaker uses a gesture. Pointing becomes important to both receptive and expressive language By the end of the naming period, the infant will use 25 words spontaneously Infants will often use an object as tool to obtain attention
Word combination period	18–24 months	Infants will combine words about 6–8 months after they say their first word If word combinations appear earlier (e.g., "let's go," "thank you"), infants are using them as a single word Holophrases also appear when the infant points to an object belonging to someone (e.g., mommy's keys) but will name the person (e.g., "mommy") as an attempt to communicate instead of "mommy's keys." This way, single words take on multiple meanings Infants typically do not combine words into phrases until their vocabulary reaches 50 words

communication can be defined as receptive, expressive, or overall language scores 1 standard deviation below the mean on standardized language tests or if articulation is unintelligible. Abnormal receptive or expressive language was based on a score of 1 SD below the mean on the receptive or expressive component of standardized language tests, respectively [69].

9.6   Proposed Interventions

We offer that there are various points during postpartum, infancy, and the early childhood years where specific interventions may be impactful in curbing potential NDI of LPIs.

9.6.1   Postpartum Period

With respect to brain development, practitioners need to have a better understanding of the cellular and molecular mechanisms that place the LPI more at risk, so that we may identify or develop and implement relevant interventions [19]. For example, LPIs' brains are not mature enough to have established mechanisms in place to protect the brain from injury caused by low blood sugar (known as hypoglycemic injury) [70, 71]. Hypoglycemia in the neonatal period is associated with injury to the brain (both white matter and gray matter injuries) [70] and specifically causes injury to the occipital region (visual processing region) in the brain leading to long-term NDI, epilepsy, and visual impairment [70, 72]. Therefore, identifying and treating hypoglycemia early are especially important.

9.6.2   Infancy

Based on the developmental phase and the NDI discussed above, early interventions are proposed but require more validation in the form of prospective studies. The early experiences that LPIs have during infancy play an important role in further developing neural circuits (i.e., nerve cell connections) [24]. This suggests that there are opportunities for intervening early to optimize brain activity during any care provided in the postnatal period and beyond.

Serve and return interactions help to build brain architecture. Serve and return interactions are based on adults responding to infant cues in a correct way. For example, when an infant or young child babbles, gestures, or cries, and an adult responds appropriately with eye contact, words, or a hug, the neural connections in the infant's brain are formed and strengthened in a way that supports the development of communication and social skills [73]. With respect to feeding, parents and caregivers need to be able to identify signs of feeding disengagement including coming off breast, pushing the artificial nipple out of mouth, pulling off the nipple, lack of active rooting or sucking, arching the back, inability to remain alert, and using a weak suck to signal the preference to return to non-nutritive sucking [72, 74, 75]. Similarly, parents should be taught that the goal of each feeding session should be an alert infant who allows for adequate intake without disorganized behavior, such as loss of milk from the sides of the mouth and pooling of milk in the mouth. Appropriate responses could include decreasing the flow of milk by adjusting the sucking burst length and respond to milk spilling out of lips with a period of rest. This will allow the infant to reorganize swallowing function [12, 72, 75]. Parents and caregivers need to be taught to identify signals of feeding distress including skin pallor, arching, limb extension, or turning away from the breast or bottle including milk spilling out of lips [76]. When parents, families, and other caregivers are sensitive to and respond to the infant's signals and needs in an appropriate way, they provide conditions that are abundant in serve and return experiences [73].

9.6.3 Early Childhood Years

We offer that multidisciplinary longitudinal follow-up clinics, specifically for the LPI population, be widely implemented to offset potential long-term NDI [56]. Multidisciplinary teams are essential in providing comprehensive anticipatory guidance-specific interventions that are critical at various developmental time frames. For example, pediatricians who attend to late preterm children should observe their language delays and make appropriate referrals to speech therapists for language development assessment and intervention [42]. There is strong evidence that shows early intervention is effective in improving cognitive outcomes for preterm children up to school age [29]. However, for interventions to be high impact, it is necessary to put a mechanism in place to identify risk factors to target those at most risk of developing neurodevelopmental delays [29]. Herein lies the direction for future research. Scholars working in this area need to come to a consensus about how such risk factors are defined and conduct research studies on which types of interventions are most useful in decreasing risks.

9.7 Limitations

Most of NDI in LPIs are based on historical cohorts. This lends the literature to observational and measurement bias. A better level of evidence is required to develop more targeted approaches to improve long-term neurodevelopmental and school-age outcomes. Therefore, LPIs need to be studied prospectively in a multidisciplinary LPIs follow-up clinic at individual hospitals. This will provide rationale for various community-based interventions.

Conclusion

The largest component of preterm infants is LPIs. This subpopulation of preterm infants is prone to experiencing developmental delay in the form of behavior, speech, and learning disorders. To promote neurodevelopment, it is critical for health-care providers, parents, and families to engage in serve and return activities. Finally, individualized care is required that includes follow-up with a multi-disciplinary team.

Take Home Messages
1. LPIs are at risk for developmental delay.
2. LPIs require longitudinal assessment from infancy to school age.
3. LPIs may experience behaviour, language, speech, and learning disorders.
4. Serve and return activities are necessary to optimize neurodevelopmental outcomes.
5. Individualized disability-based interventions are recommendations.

Appendix 1: Brain Development That Occurs in the Last Half of Gestation

- Formation of gyri and sulci
- Neurons: lamination, synaptogenesis, dendritic arborization, axonal elongation
- Oligodendrocytes: proliferation, differentiation, migration, myelin sheath synthesis
- Astrocytes: proliferation, differentiation, migration
- Microglia: proliferation, differentiation, migration [17, 25, 77–79]

Appendix 2: Explanation of Psychological Assessment Measures

18–21 Months: Psychological Assessment Measure

Bayley Scales of Infant and Toddler Development: Third Edition (Bayley–III, 2006) [80]

The Bayley Scales are standardized, individually administered assessment instruments for the evaluation of developmental functioning of infants and young children aged 1–42 months. The Bayley-III Cognitive Composite and Language Composite scores have a mean of 100, standard deviation of 15. The receptive communication and expressive communication subscales yield scores with a mean of 10 and standard deviation of 3. Reliability and validity of these instruments have been established. For example, for the Bayley-III Cognitive Composite: average reliability coefficient, $r = 0.91$; test-retest stability for ages 19–26 months, corrected $r = 0.86$; correlation with the MDI, $r = 0.60$; correlation with the Wechsler Preschool and Primary Scale of Intelligence-III Full Scale IQ, $r = 0.79$. For the Bayley-III Language Composite: average reliability coefficient, $r = 0.93$; test-retest stability for ages 33–42 months, corrected $r = 0.94$; correlation with the Preschool Language Scales (PLS-4), Language Composite, $r = 0.66$.

36 Months: School Age Psychological Assessment Measures

Wechsler Preschool and Primary Scale of Intelligence: Fourth Edition (WPPSI–IV, 2012) [81]

The WPPSI-IV measure is a standardized, individually administered clinical instrument for measuring intelligence in young children aged 2 years 6 months up to age 7 years 6 months. Full Scale Intelligence Quotients (FSIQ) have a mean of 100 and standard deviation of 15. Strong evidence for the reliability and validity of these measures are presented in detail in the technical manuals (e.g., FSIQ reliability coefficient for ages 3 years and months to 3 years and 5 months, $r = 0.95$; test-retest stability coefficient for FSIQ, corrected $r = 0.93$; correlation with the Differential Ability Scales-II General Conceptual Ability score, $r = 0.81$).

Leiter International Performance Scale: Third Edition (Leiter-3, 2013) [82]

The Leiter scale is an individually administered test for assessment of nonverbal cognitive functions in individuals aged 3 years 0 months (Leiter-3) up to adulthood. The cognitive battery yields an IQ score with a mean of 100 and standard deviation of 15. Reliability and validity statistics are reported in the test manuals (e.g., for the Leiter-3 Nonverbal IQ score: reliability for the 3–6 age group is 0.96; test-retest reliabilities for the cognitive subtests range from 0.74 to 0.86; correlation with the Stanford-Binet-5 IQ $r = 0.77$).

Adaptive Behavior Assessment System: Third Edition (ABAS-3, 2015) [83]

The ABAS assessments are rating scales completed by respondents (e.g., parents) to provide comprehensive measures of individuals' adaptive skills in conceptual, social, practical, and motor domains. The Global Assessment Composite score has a mean of 100 and standard deviation of 15. Reliability and validity measures are provided in the manual (e.g., for the ABAS-3 Parent/Primary Caregiver Form GAC: the reliability coefficient for children aged 3 years 0 months to 3 years 5 months was 0.98; test-retest reliability corrected $r = 0.82$; correlation with the Vineland-II $r = 0.77$).

Child Behavior Checklist for Ages 1½–5 (CBCL/1½–5, 2000) [84]

The CBCL is a means of obtaining standardized ratings by parents of their young children's behavioral, emotional, and social functioning. The manual reports that test-retest reliability for the internalizing scale was 0.90, externalizing scale was 0.97, and total problems were 0.90. Criterion-related validity was determined by the ability of the items to discriminate significantly between children referred for mental health or special education services and demographically similar children who were not referred. All except two of the 99 items discriminated significantly ($p < 0.01$) between the two groups.

Preschool Language Scales: Fifth Edition (PLS-5, 2011) [85]

The PLS-4 and PLS-5 measures are standardized, individually administered clinical instruments for determining language delay or disorder in children aged birth and up to age 7 years 11 months.

Total language scores, auditory comprehension scales, and expressive communication scales are norm-referenced with a mean of 100 and standard deviation of 15. The test items assess prelinguistic communication, semantics, morphology, syntax, pragmatics, and integrative language skills. Evidence for the reliability and validity of these measures are presented in detail in the technical manuals (e.g., for the PLS-5: test-retest reliability coefficient for AC for ages 3 years 0 months to 4 years 11 months, adjusted r = 0.90; correlations with the CELFP-2, range from $r = 0.70$ to 0.82).

Receptive-Expressive Emergent Language Test: Third Edition (REEL-3, 2003) [86]

The REEL is a rating scale completed by parents to provide a measure of their child's receptive, expressive, and overall language development. Children aged birth to 3 years are compared to norm-referenced samples to provide standard scores, with a mean of 100 and a standard deviation of 15. Reliability and validity statistics are reported in the test manual (e.g., for the receptive language subtest score: test-retest reliability is 0.89; correlation with the early language milestone scale—second edition $r = 0.62$).

Clinical Evaluation of Language Fundamentals Preschool Second Edition (CELFP-2, 2004) [87]

The CELFP-2 measure is a standardized, individually administered clinical instrument for determining language delay or disorder in children aged 3 years and 0 months to 6 years and 11 months. Core language scores, receptive language scores, expressive language scores, language content scores, and language structures scores are norm-referenced with a mean of 100 and standard deviation of 15. Reliability and validity measures are provided in the manual (e.g., test-retest reliability coefficient for core language score for ages 3 years and 0 months to 3 years and 11 months, adjusted $r = 0.92$; correlation with the PLS-4, range from $r = 0.73$ to 0.76).

Children's Communication Checklist Second Edition (CCC-2, 2003) [88]

The CCC-2 is a means of obtaining standardized ratings, by parents, of aspects of their child's communication that are not easy to evaluate in the traditional clinical assessment. There are ten different scales that take the context of the child's communication into account and also consider how the children use language in their various environments. For children aged 4 years and 0 months to under 16 years, scaled scores with a mean of 10 and standard deviation of 3 and percentile rank scores are calculated for each of the ten scales. A general communication competence score is calculated by comparison to a normative sample and reported in a percentile ranking. The test manual provides cutoff scores that represent the bottom 10%, 5%, and 3% of children for each 2-month age interval and reports that inter-rater reliability for ratings given by parents versus teachers/slps ranges from $r = 0.157$ for more context/environmental-driven scales to $r = 0.529$ for the more structural speech pronunciation scale. Internal consistency for each scale and predictive validity of the GCC are described in the manual.

Parent Report of Children's Abilities-Revised (PARCA-R) [89]

The Parent Report of Children's Abilities-Revised is a questionnaire-based test for assessing cognitive and language development in moderate and late preterm infants. This test has very good concurrent validity and sensitivity (90%) and specificity (76%) for detection of moderate to severe cognitive developmental delay in the moderate and late preterm infants. This test may be used as a clinical screening tool.

Photo Articulation Test (PAT-3) [90]

The PAT-3 enables professionals to assess articulation errors. The test consists of 72 photographs that test consonants and vowels. The same photographs may be used in speech-language remediation. The PAT-3 was standardized in a 23-state sample of more than 800 public and private school students in prekindergarten through grade 4. Percentiles, standard scores, and age equivalents are provided. Internal consistency, test-retest, and interscorer reliability coefficients approximate 0.80 at most ages and are in the 0.90s.

Appendix 3: Timing of Administration of Developmental Tests

See Table 9.4

Table 9.4 Common developmental tests for cognitive, language, and speech assessments at various ages

Age	Psychological and language assessment measures
18–21 months	Bayley Scales of Infant and Toddler Development: Third Edition (Bayley-III, 2006) [80]
36 months–5 years	Wechsler Preschool and Primary Scale of Intelligence: Fourth Edition (WPPSI-IV, 2012) [81]
	Leiter International Performance Scale: Third Edition (Leiter-3, 2013) [82]
	Adaptive Behavior Assessment System: Third Edition (ABAS-3, 2015) [83]
	Child Behavior Checklist for Ages 1½–5 (CBCL/1½–5, 2000) [84]
	Preschool Language Scales: Fifth Edition (PLS-5, 2011) [85]
	Receptive-Expressive Emergent Language Test: Third Edition (REEL-3, 2003) [86]
	Clinical Evaluation of Language Fundamentals Preschool Second Edition (CELFP-2, 2004) [87]
	Children's Communication Checklist Second Edition (CCC-2, 2003) [88]
	Parent Report of Children's Abilities-Revised (PARCA-R) [89]
	Photo Articulation Test (PAT-3) [90]

References

1. Allen MC, Cristofalo EA, Kim C. Outcomes of preterm infants: morbidity replaces mortality. Clin Perinatol. 2011;38:441–54.
2. Klebanoff MA, Keim SA. Epidemiology: the changing face of preterm birth. Clin Perinatol. 2011;38(3):339–50.
3. Tomashek KM, Shapiro-Mendoza CK, Davidoff MJ, Petrini JR. Differences in mortality between late-preterm and term singleton infants in the United States, 1995–2002. J Pediatr. 2007;151:450–6.
4. Khashu M, Narayanan M, Bhargava S, Osiovich H. Perinatal outcomes associated with preterm birth at 33 to 36 weeks' gestation: a population-based cohort study. Pediatrics. 2009;23:109–13.
5. Shapiro-Mendoza CK, Tomashek KM, Kotelchuck M, Barfield W, Nannini A, Weiss J, Declercq E. Effect of late-preterm birth and maternal medical conditions on newborn morbidity risk. Pediatrics. 2008;121:e223–32.
6. Visruthan NK, Agarwal P, Sriram B, Rajadurai VS. Neonatal outcome of the late preterm infant (34 to 36 Weeks): the Singapore story. Ann Acad Med Singap. 2015;44:235–43.
7. Walker M. Breastfeeding management for the late preterm infant: practical interventions for "little imposters". Clin Lact. 2010;1:22–6.
8. Medoff-Cooper B, Bilker W, Kaplan J. Sucking behavior as a function of gestational age: a cross-sectional study. Infant Behav Dev. 2001;24:83–94.
9. Bakewell-Sachs S. Near-term/late preterm infants. Newborn Infant Nurs Rev. 2007;7:68–71.

10. Laptook A, Jackson GL. Cold stress and hypoglycemia in the late preterm ("near-term") infant: impact on nursery of admission. Semin Perinatol. 2006;30:24–7.
11. The American Academy of Breastfeeding Medicine. ABM clinical protocol #10: breastfeeding the late preterm infant (340/7–366/7 weeks gestation) (first revision June 2011). Breastfeed Med. 2011;6:151–6.
12. Baker B. Evidence-based practice to improve outcomes for late preterm infants. J Obstet Gynecol Neonatal Nurs. 2015;44:127–34.
13. Gouyon JB, Iacobelli S, Ferdynus C, Bonsante F. Neonatal problems of late and moderate preterm infants. Semin Fetal Neonatal Med. 2012;17:146–52.
14. Wang ML, Dorer DJ, Fleming MP, Catlin EA. Clinical outcomes of near-term infants. Pediatrics. 2004;114:372–6.
15. Hillman N. Hyperbilirubinemia in the late preterm infant. Newborn Infant Nurs Rev. 2007;7:91–4.
16. Walsh JM, Doyle LW, Anderson PJ, Lee KJ, Cheong JL. Moderate and late preterm birth: effect on brain size and maturation at term-equivalent age. Radiology. 2014;273(1): 232–40.
17. Munakata S, Okada T, Okahashi A, et al. Gray matter volumetric MRI differences late-preterm and term infants. Brain and Development. 2013;35:10–6.
18. Kinney HC. The near-term (late preterm) human brain and risk for periventricular leukomalacia: a review. Semin Perinatol. 2006;30:81–8.
19. Billiards SS, Pierson CR, Haynes RL, Folkerth RD, Kinney HC. Is the late preterm infant more vulnerable to gray matter injury than the term infant? Clin Perinatol. 2006;33:915–33.
20. Kugelman A, Colin AA. Late preterm infants: near term but still in a critical developmental time period. Pediatrics. 2013;132:741–51.
21. Mally PV, Bailey S, Hendricks-Muñoz KD. Clinical issues in the management of late preterm infants. Curr Probl Pediatr Adolesc Health Care. 2010;40:218–33.
22. Hüppi PS, Warfield S, Kikinis R, Barnes PD, Zientara GP, Jolesz FA, Tsuji MK, Volpe JJ. Quantitative magnetic resonance imaging of brain development in premature and mature newborns. Ann Neurol. 1998;43:224–35.
23. Benders MJ, Palmu K, Menache C, Borradori-Tolsa C, Lazeyras F, Sizonenko S, Dubois J, Vanhatalo S, Hüppi PS. Early brain activity relates to subsequent brain growth in premature infants. Cereb Cortex. 2014;25(9):3014–24.
24. Tau GZ, Peterson BS. Normal development of brain circuits. Neuropsychopharmacology. 2010;35:3014–24.
25. Kelly CE, Cheong JL, Fam LG, Leemans A, Seal ML, Doyle LW, Anderson PJ, Spittle AJ, Thompson DK. Moderate and late preterm infants exhibit widespread brain white matter microstructure alterations at term-equivalent age relative to term-born controls. Brain Imaging Behav. 2016;10:41–9.
26. Kapellou O, Counsell SJ, Kennea N, Dyet L, Saeed N, Stark J, Maalouf E, Duggan P, Ajayi-Obe M, Hajnal J, Allsop JM. Abnormal cortical development after premature birth shown by altered allometric scaling of brain growth. PLoS Med. 2006;3:1382–90.
27. Raju TN. The "Late preterm" birth – ten years later. Pediatr. 2017;139:e20163331.
28. Vohr B. Long-term outcomes of moderately preterm, late preterm, and early term infants. Clin Perinatol. 2013;40:739–51.
29. Cheong JL, Doyle LW, Burnett AC, Lee KJ, Walsh JM, Potter CR, Treyvaud K, Thompson DK, Olsen JE, Anderson PJ, Spittle AJ. Association between moderate and late preterm birth and neurodevelopment and social-emotional development at age 2 years. JAMA Pediatr. 2017;171:e164805.
30. Lunsing RJ. Subtle bilirubin-induced neurodevelopmental dysfunction (BIND) in the term and late preterm infant: does it exist? Semin Perinatol. 2014;38:465–71.
31. Johnson L, Bhutani VK. The clinical syndrome of bilirubin-induced neurologic dysfunction. Semin Perinatol. 2011;35:101–13.
32. Watchko JF. Hyperbilirubinemia and bilirubin toxicity in the late preterm infant. Clin Perinatol. 2006;33:839–52.

33. Volpe J. Neurology of the newborn. 5th ed. Philadelphia, PA: Saunders Elsevier; 2008. p. 619–51.
34. Romeo DM, Ricci D, Brogna C, Cilauro S, Lombardo ME, Romeo MG, et al. Neurological examination of late-preterm infants at term age. Eur J Paediatr Neurol. 2011;15:353–60.
35. Ricci D, Romeo DM, Haataja L, van Haastert IC, Cesarini L, Maunu J, et al. Neurological examination of preterm infants at term equivalent age. Early Hum Dev. 2008;84:751–61.
36. Morse SB, Zheng H, Tang Y, Roth J. Early school-age outcomes of late preterm infants. Pediatrics. 2009;123(4):e622–9.
37. Romeo D, Cioni M, Scoto M, Palermo F, Romeo M, Mercuri E. Application of a scorable neurologic examination to near-term infants: longitudinal data. Neuropediatrics. 2007;38:1–6.
38. Prins SA, von Lindern JS, van Dijk S, Versteegh FG. Motor development of premature infants born between 32 and 34 weeks. Int J Pediatr. 2010;2010:462048. https://doi.org/10.1155/2010/462048.
39. Woythaler MA, McCormick MC, Smith VC. Late preterm infants have worse 24-month neurodevelopmental outcomes than term infants. Pediatrics. 2011;127:e622–9.
40. Johnson S, Evans TA, Draper ES, Field DJ, Manktelow BN, Marlow N, et al. Neurodevelopmental outcomes following late and moderate prematurity: a population-based cohort study. Arch Dis Child Fetal Neonatal Ed. 2015;100:F301–8.
41. Spittle AJ, Walsh JM, Potter C, Mcinnes E, Olsen JE, Lee KJ, et al. Neurobehaviour at term-equivalent age and neurodevelopmental outcomes at 2 years in infants born moderate-to-late preterm. Dev Med Child Neurol. 2017;59:207–15.
42. Putnick DL, Bornstein MH, Eryigit-Madzwamuse S, Wolke D. Long-term stability of language performance in very preterm, moderate-late preterm, and term children. J Pediatr. 2017;181:74–9.
43. Cheong JL, Thompson DK, Spittle AJ, Potter CR, Walsh JM, Burnett AC, et al. Brain volumes at term-equivalent age are associated with 2-year neurodevelopment in moderate and late preterm children. J Pediatr. 2016;174:91–7.
44. Stene-Larsen K, Brandlistuen RE, Lang AM, Landolt MA, Latal B, Vollrath ME. Communication impairments in early term and late preterm children: a prospective cohort study following children to age 36 months. J Pediatr. 2014;165:1123–8.
45. Rabie NZ, Bird TM, Magann EF, Hall RW, McKelvey SS. ADHD and developmental speech/language disorders in late preterm, early term and term infants. J Perinatol. 2015;35:660–4.
46. Baron IS, Erickson K, Ahronovich MD, Baker R, Litman FR. Cognitive deficit in preschoolers born late-preterm. Early Hum Dev. 2011;87:115–9.
47. Talge NM, Holzman C, Wang J, et al. Late-preterm birth and its association with cognitive and socioemotional outcomes at 6 years of age. Pediatrics. 2010;126:1124–31.
48. McGowan JE, Alderdice FA, Holmes VA, Johnston L. Early childhood development of late-preterm infants: a systematic review. Pediatrics. 2011;127:1111–24.
49. Boyle JD, Boyle EM. Born just a few weeks early: does it matter? Arch Dis Child Fetal Neonatal Ed. 2013;98:F85–8.
50. Moster D, Lie RT, Markestad T. Long-term medical and social consequences of preterm birth. N Engl J Med. 2008;359:262–73.
51. Petrini JR, Dias T, McCormick MC, et al. Increased risk of adverse neurological development for late preterm infants. J Pediatr. 2009;154:169–76.
52. Hirvonen M, Ojala R, Korhonen P, et al. Cerebral palsy among children born moderately and late preterm. Pediatrics. 2014;134:e1584–93.
53. Chan E, Quigley MA. School performance at age 7 years in late preterm and early term birth: a cohort study. Arch Dis Child Fetal Neonatal Ed. 2014;99:F451–7.
54. Quigley MA, Poulsen G, Boyle E, et al. Early term and late preterm birth are associated with poorer school performance at age 5 years: a cohort study. Arch Dis Child Fetal Neonatal Ed. 2012;97:F167–73.
55. Peacock PJ, Henderson J, Odd D, Emond A. Early school attainment in late-preterm infants. Arch Dis Child. 2012;97(2):118–20.

56. Chyi LJ, Lee HC, Hintz SR, Gould JB, Sutcliffe TL. School outcomes of late preterm infants: special needs and challenges for infants born at 32 to 36 weeks gestation. J Pediatr. 2008;153:25–31.
57. Jain L. School outcome in late preterm infants: a cause for concern. J Pediatr. 2008;153:5–6.
58. Lipkind HS, Slopen ME, Pfeiffer MR, McVeigh KH. School-age outcomes of late preterm infants in New York City. Am J Obstet Gynecol. 2012;206:e221–6.
59. MacKay DF, Smith GC, Dobbie R, Pell JP. Gestational age at delivery and special educational need: retrospective cohort study of 407,503 school children. PLoS Med. 2010;7:e1000289.
60. Gray RF, Indurkhya A, McCormick MC. Prevalence, stability, and predictors of clinically significant behavior problems in low birth weight children at 3, 5, and 8 years of age. Pediatrics. 2004;114:736–43.
61. McCormick MC, Workman-Daniels K, Brooks-Gunn J. The behavioral and emotional well-being of school-age children with different birth weights. Pediatrics. 1996;97:18–25.
62. Lindstrom K, Winbladh B, Haglund B, Hjern A. Preterm infants as young adults: a Swedish national cohort study. Pediatrics. 2007;120:70–7.
63. de Jong M, Verhoeven M, van Baar AL. School outcome, cognitive functioning, and behaviour problems in moderate and late preterm children and adults: a review. Semin Fetal Neonatal Med. 2012;17:163–9.
64. Harris MN, Voigt RG, Barbaresi WJ, et al. ADHD and learning disabilities in former late preterm infants: a population-based birth cohort. Pediatrics. 2013;132:e630–6.
65. Odd DE, Lingam R, Emond A, Whitelaw A. Movement outcomes of infants born moderate and late preterm. Acta Paediatr. 2013;102:876–82.
66. Synnes A, Luu TM, Moddemann D, Church P, Lee D, Vincer M, Ballantyne M, et al. Determinants of developmental outcomes in a very preterm Canadian cohort. Arch Dis Child Fetal Neonatal Ed. 2017;102:F235–4.
67. Russman BS, Gage JR. Cerebral palsy. Curr Probl Pediatr. 1989;19:65–111.
68. Palisano R, Rosenbaum P, Walter S, Russell D, Wood E, Galuppi B. Development and reliability of a system to classify gross motor function in children with cerebral palsy. Dev Med Child Neurol. 1997;39:214–23.
69. Johnson CP, Blasco PA. Infant growth and development. Pediatr Rev. 1997;18(7):224–42.
70. Garg M, Devaskar SU. Glucose metabolism in the late preterm infant. Clin Perinatol. 2006;33:853–70.
71. Cornblath M, Ichord R. Hypoglycemia in the neonate. Semin Perinatol. 2000;14:136–49.
72. Tam EW, Haeusslein LA, Bonifacio SL, Glass HC, Rogers EE, Jeremy RJ, Barkovich AJ, Ferriero DM. Hypoglycemia is associated with increased risk for brain injury and adverse neurodevelopmental outcome in neonates at risk for encephalopathy. J Pediatr. 2012;161:88–93.
73. Center on the Developing Child at Harvard University. From best practices to breakthrough impacts: a science-based approach to building a more promising future for young children and families. 2016. http://www.developingchild.harvard.edu
74. Shaker C. Nipple feeding preterm infants: an individualized, developmentally supportive approach. Neonatal Netw. 1999;18:15–22.
75. Dosani A, Currie G. Supporting public health nurses with breastfeeding interventions for late preterm infants. Austin Pediatr. 2017;4:1057.
76. Thompson DG. Focusing on feeding skills evaluating inadequate weight gain in late preterm infants. Infant Child Adolesc Nutr. 2010;2:147–51.
77. Lan LM, Yamashita Y, Tang Y, Sugahara T, Takahashi M, Ohba T, Okamura H. Normal fetal brain development: MR imaging with a half-fourier rapid acquisition with relaxation enhancement sequence. Radiology. 2000;215(1):205–10.
78. Darnall RA, Ariagno RL, Kinney HC. The late preterm infant and the control of breathing, sleep, and brainstem development: a review. Clin Perinatol. 2006;33:883–914.
79. Delaney AL, Arvedson JC. Development of swallowing and feeding: prenatal through first year of life. Dev Disabil Res Rev. 2008;14:105–17.
80. Bayley N. Bayley scales of infant and toddler development. 3rd ed. San Antonio, TX: Harcourt Assessment, Inc; 2006.

81. Wechsler D. Wechsler preschool and primary scale of intelligence. 4th ed. Bloomington, MN: Pearson; 2012.
82. Roid G, Miller L, Pomplun M, Koch C. Leiter international performance scale. Wood Dale, IL: Stoelting; 2013.
83. Harrison P, Oakland T. Adaptive behavior assessment system. 3rd ed. Terrance, CA: WPS; 2015.
84. Achenbach TM, Rescorla LA. Manual for the ASEBA preschool forms & profiles. Burlington, VT: University of Vermont, Research Center for Children, Youth, & Families; 2000.
85. Zimmerman I, Steiner V, Pond R. Preschool language scales. PLS-5 manual. 5th ed. Bloomington, MN: NCS Pearson, Inc; 2011.
86. Bzoch K, League R, Brown V. Receptive-expressive emergent language test. Third edition. REEL 3 manual. Austin, TX: Pro-ed Inc; 2003.
87. Wiig E, Secord W, Semel E. Clinical evaluation of language fundamentals preschool – second edition. CELF-P2 manual. San Antonio, TX: Harcourt Assessment Inc; 2004.
88. Bishop DVM. The children's communication checklist, 2nd ed. CCC-2 manual. London: The Psychological Corporation; 2003.
89. Blaggan S, Guy A, Boyle EM, Spata E, Manktelow BN, Wolke D, Johnson S. A parent questionnaire for developmental screening in infants born late and moderately preterm. Pediatrics. 2014;134:e55–62.
90. Lippke B, Dickey S, Selmar J, Soder A. Photo articulation test. Third edition. PAT-3 manual. In: Inc. Austin, TX: Pro-ed; 1997.

Perspectives from Health-Care Providers Local to Global: Words of Wisdom— Personal Reflections on Caring for Late Preterm Infants

10

Carole Kenner and Shahirose Sadrudin Premji

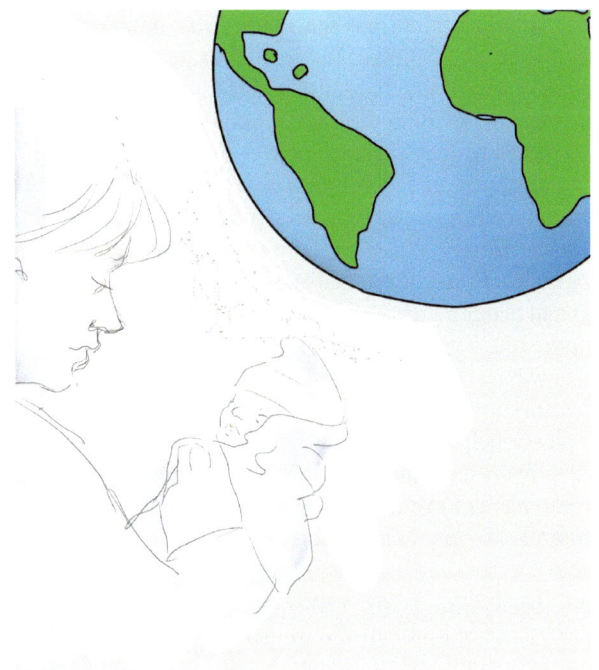

C. Kenner (✉)
School of Nursing and Health and Exercise Science, The College of New Jersey, New York, NY, USA

Council of International Neonatal Nurses, Inc. (COINN), Yardley, PA, USA

S. S. Premji
School of Nursing, Faculty of Health, York University, Toronto, ON, Canada
e-mail: premjis@yorku.ca

Late preterm infants and their families require recognition that their needs are different from the very preterm or term infant and family. Globally care for this population varies widely. This chapter brings together personal perspectives that present LPIs within a country context and health-care professionals' personal stories of providing care to this vulnerable population. Narratives from Brazil, Japan, Malawi, Russia, and South Africa weave the collective story.

Our first story is from the state of Hawaii. In this culture, family is a very important concept and member of the care team. The rate of preterm births in 2013 was 9.1% of all live births or 1 in 11 [1].

Hawai'i: Susan Kau, RNC-NIC, Staff Nurse, Kapi'olani Medical Center for Women and Children, Honolulu, Hawai'i

We are a unique population—medical and textbooks categorize us as the 34 0/7– 36 6/7 weekers. Other terms used to describe us are near term and moderate preterm. The late preterm infants are the new "baby boomers" in our NICU. We outnumber the patient population of micropremies, term, and post-term infants. We have a higher risk of morbidity, mortality and readmission rates due to dehydration, hyperbilirubinemia, and feeding difficulties to name a few.

Our clinical problems may include some or all of the following: respiratory distress, apnea, bradycardia and desaturations also known as A/B/Ds, temperature instability, hypoglycemia, hyperbilirubinemia, as well as being "problematic" breast and bottle feeders.

Respiratory issues: Some of us need assistance after birth to breathe. New words for our parents and in our own vocabulary include oxygen, ventilator, nasal intermittent positive pressure ventilation (NIPPV), continuous positive airway pressure (CPAP), high-flow nasal cannula (HFNC), low-flow nasal cannula (LFNC), surfactant, apnea, desaturations, pulse oximetry, and caffeine to name a few. One request we have is to please help us to rest and grow by positioning us comfortably using developmental support aids and guidelines. Please share the benefits of kangaroo care with my parents and encourage my mom and dad to do kangaroo care when they are visiting us. We appreciate "quiet times" as well as having our cares and exams clustered.

Temperature instability: We are especially vulnerable to hypothermia that can lead to a whole cascade of problems for us including increased oxygen consumption that can lead to hypoxia, increased glucose utilization, and depletion of glycogen stores that can lead to hypoglycemia. More new words to learn here is incubator (isolette), servocontrol skin probe (ISC) vs neutral thermal environment (NTE) mode, and bassinet to crib. Since we are not quite term, we lack enough brown fat (substance that is accumulated in increasing amounts as the infant advances through gestation). Please help us conserve our body heat by helping maintain a normal body temperature. Another benefit of kangaroo care is here. The next step for us is "wean to crib." This is a period of time when we are trending adequate weight gain with less to no support from our incubators. We now graduate, so we can wear clothes, be swaddled, and be placed in a bassinet. One step closer to home. Yeah!!

Feeding issues: Bottle and breastfeeding seems to be the biggest hurdle for us. We are often referred to as "wimps" and "poky eaters." Terms in our vocabulary include gavage feeds with nasogastric tube (NGT) or orogastric tube (OGT) and fortifying for calories from 22 up to 27 calories to help us with weight gain. We start with trophic feeds (small amounts that are enough to tickle our throats) every 4 h then progress to every 3 h. The volumes are calculated based on our weights and total fluids that the medical team decides for us. Can you believe that some of us only get as little as 1 teaspoon (5 cc) every 4 h to start!! The next step is bottle-feeding which is something that term babies don't seem to have a problem with. We need slow flow nipples (many different brands—some try many before settling on the right one); we need pacing (the mnemonic—suck, swallow, breathe), the side-lying position, and a speech therapist to help.

Hyperbilirubinemia: The key word here is to educate my family (especially first-time mothers) on how to evaluate feedings and what signs to look for to detect dehydration and jaundice.

We offer challenges like no other in terms of timing of our discharge. Although some of us are larger (large for gestational age, LGA) than someone else with our same gestation (small for gestational age, SGA, or average for gestational age, AGA), we are not all the same!! We are all individuals with different names and personalities. Just remember, "we call the shots!!". It is not uncommon for us to try the "patience" of our caregivers (medical doctors, nurses, physical therapists, occupational therapists, speech therapists, and especially our parents who want us home). During am medical rounds, please call us by our first names—it makes us feel special.

Our parents/caregivers absolutely need to be equipped to work with and against any disadvantages that might come with the way we are categorized by our birth. Arguably we that are born into the less-empowered categories need parents/caregivers to be particularly mindful of upcoming challenges. The world is our oyster!!

Our next story is from the state of Tennessee by a Japanese-American nurse. In 2012 the percentage of late preterm births in Tennessee was estimated to be between 7.8% and 8.1% [2].

Tennessee: Wakako Eklund, DNP, APN, NNP-BC, Neonatal Nurse Practitioner, Pediatrix, Nashville, TN, Adjunct Faculty, College of Engineering & Science-Louisiana Tech University, Rushton, LA

A 34-week male infant was born to a well-educated mother who took excellent care of herself throughout her pregnancy. The parents and his older brother with utmost delight as well as anticipation for their future life together as a family of four welcomed the baby. The baby's lungs, however, began to show signs of distress. The little infant developed respiratory distress syndrome and was unable to conquer the battle. Further complications led to development of devastating necrotizing enterocolitis, disseminated intravascular coagulation, and multi-organ failure. The baby boy passed away after 59 days, leaving the family devastated, even the older brother who was in kindergarten at the time who was left deeply affected by this loss in an unimaginable way. This was in 1971 in well-developed country, however, before the availability of surfactant and antenatal steroids. This was my first encounter with a loss of an infant and he was a late preterm infant. He was my dear cousin. I came to have a much deeper appreciation for the risks that late preterm infants are exposed to even in the era of surfactant and antenatal steroids. It was not until I stepped foot in the neonatal world that I fully understood what occurred to my cousin and his family, not only physiologically but also psychosocially.

Today's late preterm infants are born with a much higher likelihood of "making it" without any life-altering issues, thanks to the advanced understanding of neonatal physiology as well as the availability of treatment. However, we cannot overlook the risks that these infants face. Evidence is now available to increase the awareness of the risks for late preterm infants including the need for vigilance in monitoring respiratory status, vital signs, blood glucose levels, bilirubin levels, or feeding tolerance. In addition, bonding is challenged; attainment of direct breastfeeding is also a significant hurdle for these infants.

I personally experienced caring for numbers of late preterm infants throughout my professional life as a neonatal nurse practitioner. I have seen those who did not survive the stressful delivery even after timely resuscitation efforts. Many developed complications of respiratory distress leading to irreparable damage. Certainly, the number of successful discharges of late preterm infants outnumbers those who face complications; however, late preterm infants do face serious challenges.

My encounter with families who are about to deliver late preterm infants begins with explaining to them that their infants are not "almost term," but they are "late preterm." Many clinical sites have admission orders that address the need to recognize and prevent hypoglycemia or to provide additional observation for these infants. We must remember, however, that we have mothers arriving at the obstetrical triage whose infants' gestational ages may not be clearly established due to limited prenatal care or a lack of prenatal records at the time of the birth. It is always helpful to provide verbal reminders to the staff members to ensure that even the newest nursing staff is made aware of the risks that these infants face so that we do not care for the infants as if they are "almost term." Parents observe how the healthcare team demonstrates our concern and translates our knowledge into care.

My personal approach is not to overwhelm the family with all the potential risks at the time of the initial encounter but to gradually add information to ensure that family members are not blindsided when certain conditions develop. For example, I may casually describe the potential need for respiratory support and for vigilance in monitoring the feeding efforts or blood glucose level. However, if the infants exhibit respiratory conditions that are more than transitional respiratory distress and are placed on supportive devices, such as continuous airway positive pressure (CPAP) or high-flow nasal cannula (HFNC), then, I begin to fine-tune associated risks and conditions that I would like them to be made aware of. Delayed feeding due to the invasive respiratory support may immediately alert us of the need to further discuss the potential delays in attainment of full feeding, development of hyperbilirubinemia, and of frequent challenges with oral feeding vs tube feeding, or development of feeding intolerance. I find it effective to gradually increase the details of current and potential challenges while strongly supporting their role as partners in care. Parents' loving presence, an integrated presence, to be available for their infants to perform daily care and provide skin-to-skin care or kangaroo mother care cannot be replaced with any advanced medical care. We must make sure that the family members are aware of their importance while learning of the challenges that their infants are facing.

When the complications are highly challenging, my personal knowledge of the psychosocial and emotional challenges that parents and siblings live with throughout their lives always remains with me. The care and concerns for the late preterm infants and their families may not significantly differ from that of the care for much smaller infants. The fact that the parents enter our area feeling that "our babies are almost term" instead of "our babies may be barely viable" creates a difference in the mindset of the family that leads to the unique needs and requires sensitivity to these differences.

The next story comes from Russia. The rate of late preterm births is not reported; however, the rate of preterm births is 7.0% or 7/100 live births in 2010 [3].

Russia: Marina Boykova, PhD, RN, Assistant Professor, Holy Family University, Philadelphia, PA and Board of Director-at Large, Council of International Neonatal Nurses, Inc. (COINN)

The baby born between 34 and 36 weeks of gestation posed no perceived risks when I began my nursing career almost 30 years ago in Russia. I worked in a tertiary center in large city in Russia. The care rarely differed from term baby care. Yet, these babies often seem to have some characteristics resembling a preterm infant that is born before 34 weeks of gestation. This statement may sound strange as the accepted definition of prematurity is born before 37 weeks of gestation, but many parents and health professionals did not consider the late preterm infant as premature. Through time and research, we now know these babies have immature brain development, as the brain and central nervous system are the fastest growing system at that gestational age. These babies are not just term babies born a little early. They are preterm infants and need to be assessed and treated as immature babies.

The next story is from Malawi where in 2010, the rate of prematurity was estimated to be 18% [4].

Malawi: Prof. Address Malata, PhD, MScN, Pricipal of Kamuzu College of Nursing, University of Malawi, President of the Association of Malawian Midwives, Vice-President, International Council of Midwives and Prof. Wilson Mandala, PhD, Senior Researcher and Acting Executive Dean, Malawi University of Science and Technology, Malawi

Late preterm infants often have the same size and weight of some term infants (those born at 37–41 weeks of gestation); it is very easy for parents, caregivers, and health-care professionals to erroneously treat them as though they are developmentally mature and at low risk of morbidity.

With a per capita income of US$290 per year and 80% of its population living in rural areas, Malawi is considered one of the poorest countries [5]. Malawi also has one of the highest estimated neonatal mortality rate, estimated to be 33 per every 1000 live births. This high neonatal mortality rate is thought to be partly a result of Malawi also having one of the highest rates of preterm birth in the world with nearly 1 in 5 babies born before 37 weeks of gestation [6].

Both the public and private sectors provide Malawi's health services. Only four central hospitals are adequately equipped to ably and satisfactorily handle late preterm babies. The current practices that are used in these hospitals include the following, which are also in line with the current WHO recommendations [7]. Antenatally, these measures include use of antenatal corticosteroids, provision of magnesium sulfate for fetal protection against neurological complications, administrations of antibiotics especially erythromycin, but not the combination of amoxicillin and clavulanic acid, "co-amoxiclav" for some but not all women in preterm labor. The message we want to convey for health professionals caring for the late preterm infant involves thermal care—continuous kangaroo mother care (KMC) in the stable infant and mother [8]. Where continuous KMC is not possible, such as where the mother had a C-section, then intermittent KMC is recommended. Those preterm infants not on continuous or intermittent KMC should be cared for in a thermoneutral environment either under radiant warmers or in an incubator. Unfortunately in our country, this equipment is not always available. Late preterm infants who are diagnosed with respiratory disorder syndrome are supposed to be put on continuous positive airway pressure (CPAP) therapy as soon as the diagnosis is made. In low-resourced countries like ours, a low-cost bubble CPAP is a possible alternative. Surfactant replacement therapy is not recommended as a prophylaxis in the late preterm infant with respiratory distress syndrome. Oxygen therapy is needed in some of the late preterm infants. Most if not all of these services are only available for babies born in urban areas, which is less than 20% of the total population. Those born in rural areas would have to travel long distances to primary and secondary tier health facilities that might not have any of these facilities. The way forward therefore is for the Malawi government to make most of these measures and interventions available in all health facilities in the country especially those in the rural areas as laid out in its strategic plans for the next 5 years.

The following story comes from Zambia where the late preterm infant birth rate reported in 2010 was 13/100 live births [9].

Zambia: Bupe Mwamba, RN, RM, School of Child and Adolescent Health, University of Cape Town, Cape Town, South Africa

My journey as a neonatal nurse started in 2006 at the completion of the 6-month internship, internship undertaken by all general registered nurses from Lusaka Schools of Nursing and Midwifery based at University Teaching Hospital (UTH) in Lusaka, Zambia. I really did not understand why I was sent to the neonatal intensive care unit (NICU) after I completed my internship. I wanted to swap to be in the main intensive care unit (MICU) for adults, but the swapping failed. That marked the beginning of a very fulfilling journey of caring for newborn babies at UTH.

UTH is the largest referral hospital in Zambia. This NICU is the only third level NICU in Zambia. Prematurity accounts for about 27.2% of all neonatal deaths in Zambia [10]. Working in the third level NICU as a newly qualified general RN was challenging at the beginning because it was a job on training. Despite having had work experience in the NICU both as a student nurse and as an intern nurse, being a full-time neonatal nurse was a different situation. One thing that I appreciated was the orientation from the then ward manager and how she allocated staff per shift. She ensured that every shift was well balanced by staff with different strengths. For example, a shift will have a nurse who is good at newborn intubation, resuscitation, and cannulation, which was an excellent staff allocation.

Zambia has three nursing shifts, that is, morning shift from 7:30 am to 1 pm, 1 pm to 6 pm, and 6 pm to 7:30 am. Being the largest NICU, the total number of patients per day ranged between 50 and 80. We used to be five to ten nurses per shift in my early years of working in NICU, which later reduced to 3–5 nurses as years went by. It was an awesome and fulfilling experience, which has led to the growth of my passion for babies and prompted me to go into midwifery, as it is the only specialty close to neonatal care.

The late preterm infant requires special attention as I learned through experience. Usually the prognosis for these babies is good. My role in the care of late preterm babies was to uphold high levels of infection prevention. Infection prevention is key in newborn care because these babies are prone to infections related to immature immune systems. Infection prevention starts at the receiving of the newborn baby from the midwife. Preparation for an admission is key; therefore at every discharge, I used to enjoy disinfecting and thoroughly cleaning of incubators and cot beds.

The motivation to do my work diligently was ignited by the area manager whose words of orientation I embedded in the apex of my heart. She said, "When a nurse working in NICU is told that her child will be admitted to NICU from the labor ward because of the condition of the baby at birth, most of them burst into tears. They know that it is a hub of infection. Therefore, as you start your work, take care of these babies as you would love your own babies to be cared for." I took these words of wisdom at heart and executed my duties with joy. I was chosen as an infection prevention (IP) liaison officer. I performed my IP duties diligently, which led into NICU's winning of the hospital award on IP. It is the passion within that has driven me into pursuing further studies in midwifery and neonatal science, and I'm now specializing in maternal and child health as I aspire to be a mentor in maternal and child health. The other aspect, which is key in the management of these babies, is the close monitoring of intravenous fluid administration because any fluid over-load is detrimental and can lead to death.

Caring for neonates is my passion and requires critical thinking, sound judgment, and excellent observational skills in the rendering quality of care. Everything is dependent on see, judge, and act because neonates cannot speak. For example, these infants are prone to necrotizing enterocolitis (NEC). To prevent NEC, one word that I will never forget is "priming" of the gut before introduction of full feeds. Priming the gut is the introduction of feeds such as expressed breastmilk at the lowest level to assess how the neonate will tolerate the feed. Thereafter a gradual increase to full feeds within a week of commencement of feeding is done.

One thing that is key in newborn care is the inner drive, which ignites the passion to do my best for these innocent souls. My self-actualization is attained through the help I render to others. What is life if not leaved for others? What legacy will you leave behind in your practice as a nurse? I have chosen mine and I will work toward being that change that people long to see in the world.

Brazil brings us the next story. The rate of late preterm births varies across the country with a reported rate in the south of 11.0% in 2004 with a rate of 10.6% in São Paulo in 2010 [11].

Brazil: Marcia Maria Tavares Machado, Nurse, Dean of Extension Federal University of Ceará, Brazil

In the 1980s, exclusive breastfeeding rates in Brazil, and especially in the Northeast, were very low, and children died of malnutrition, diarrhea, and respiratory problems. At that time, in every thousand children who were born, 95 died before completing 1 year of life. During my training in nursing in the 1980s, I started monitoring mothers and children in the maternity ward and at home helping to ensure that breastfeeding was performed in a more relaxed way and encouraging the mothers to exclusively breastfeed the babies until their 6 months of life. Many of these children who were born at the maternity school were premature—many late preterm, and this problem was a great challenge because they spent many days in the NICU.

We started a breastfeeding program at the maternity school to work with the mothers and the professionals. We instructed the mothers to milk their breasts during the period of hospitalization, and we taught the professionals to offer milk through a tube, cup, or spoon. This was one of the first challenges, because the professionals used the bottle to offer milk. We trained the nurses to do cup feedings. Initially there was a lot of resistance, although the adoption of these new practices was a priority to the director of maternity school and the nursing head, who requested the participation of the whole team in the 40-h training, with theoretical and practical classes in breastfeeding counseling.

Mothers who stayed rooming-in or returned to maternity every day were instructed to take milk out every 3 h and store it in a refrigerator or freezer, which would then be transported to the nursery for the baby. On a daily basis, the team and the mother evaluated the possibility of introducing the infant to the breast. During the NICU stay, mothers were prepared to take the baby home. The Health System (SUS) in Brazil has a home visit for all children after hospital discharge. Premature including late preterm infants are given more special care because mothers feel more insecure, and many children return to hospital after hospital discharge (with pneumonia, aspiration, otitis media, and sometimes malnutrition). Follow-up is very important, especially to support the mother to breastfeed her child. Rates of early weaning are very common in late preterm infants, and it is important to monitor the mother and child binomial.

There are several recommendations to facilitate breastfeeding the late preterm infant. They include:

- To follow the first moments of breastfeeding, the professional must have a lot of patience, technical ability, and communication skills to build a trusting, empathetic relationship with the mother and promote infant safety.
- Many late premature infants are drowsy, they take too long to suck, and this can be a deciding factor in assessing whether sucking alone is sufficient for the child to be well fed. Sometimes it is necessary to milk the breast infant and offer, after sucking at the breast, this milk in the cup, spoon, or dropper. It is very important to observe if the late premature baby is gaining weight and has a good urination (at least six times a day) to ensure adequate growth.
- When the premature baby does not gain weight, it is important for the nurse or health agent to guide the mother to offer the later breast milk (which has a higher

concentration of fat), after the baby completes the feeding, to stimulate the child to have a better gain of weight. Only when several attempts have been made and the weight does not increase should one opt for the infantile formula for the premature.

- Sometimes the mother's nipple is large or flat, and it is necessary to soften the areola and nipple before feeding to facilitate the baby's latch on the breasts.
- Using different ways to place the baby close to the breast can also be tested. Many mothers feel safer when they put their baby's body on pillow, holding the child's head with a hand. Always during the first feedings, it is important to have a well-trained professional, close to the binomial mother and child.
- A very effective strategy to prepare home environment for the late premature baby is to involve other family members, especially the father and grandmother, to receive guidance and participate in this time of breastfeeding. A family orientation protocol should be established during the hospital stay and several days prior to discharge.
- During the first months, it is important to monitor the weight every 2 weeks, and whenever possible, the nurse or community health agent should perform a home visit to evaluate the child's feedings and development.
- Due to the exchange of ideas and joint decision-making, the teamwork makes the late preterm follow-up process easier and more successful.

There are many uncertainties related to breastfeeding of late premature infants and the time of introduction of new foods to them. This evidences the need of the health services and professionals to involve the late premature babies' families in continuous education to make them autonomous while promoting effective and safe care.

Our final story is from South Africa where eight out of every ten infants are born premature [12].

South Africa: Dr. C.M. Maree, Fellow, Academy of Nursing of South Africa & Senior Lecturer, University of Pretoria, South Africa, and Dr. C. van Heerden, University of Pretoria, South Africa

In the case of the late preterm infant, the magical moment for bonding and attachment at birth might turn into a non-magical moment if the mother and baby are separated. Even if this magical moment is missed, it does not necessarily mean that bonding and attachment are lost. Bonding and attachment entail a long-term process and luckily not a single moment. It follows a predictive sequence, running parallel with physical, social, emotional, and cognitive development. The tempo, pattern, and style vary for each baby and can be influenced by being born prematurely. The sequence of bonding and attachment follow a pattern of acquisition (sensory input and short-term memory in the cortex), consolidation (transferring of information to the amygdala/emotional brain), and memory formation (storing in the frontal brain, contributing to personality formation). Attachment serves as a driving force for social, emotional, and cognitive development and future relationship. For mothers of late preterm infants, attachment and bonding may be disrupted due to the baby's need for a NICU stay away from the mother and the mother's inability to read the sometimes diverse or vague infant cues.

In our experience we have found that nurses can foster the mother-infant relationship and promote bonding and attachment. Bond and attachment are enhanced through experiences of positive sensory stimuli. Positive sensory stimuli include feeling warmth and skin-to-skin contact, the smell of the mother and her breastmilk, the taste of breastmilk, dimmed lights, and the mother's voice and her protective behavior. Nurses can help the mother recognize the importance of these stimuli as well as learn how to decrease negative ones—bright lights, noise, cold environment, overstimulation of oral senses, strong smells, and painful interventions.

The late preterm baby's long-term survival depends on attachment that might be interrupted, but parents and health-care providers can create magical moments through positive stimuli. Attachment and bonding are central to positive growth and development and a strong mother-infant relationship.

Conclusion

This chapter presents stories from around the world. Late preterm infants require special care—they are not full-term infant nor are they very, very immature, but they are vulnerable. Lessons learned and perspectives presented offer guidance on how to promote positive mother-infant interactions and infant development.

References

1. March of Dimes (MOD). Born too soon and too small in Hawaii. 2015. Available from: https://www.marchofdimes.org/peristats/pdflib/195/15.pdf.
2. Centers for Disease Control & Prevention (CDC). *QuickStats*: Percentage of Infants Born Late Preterm, * by Mother's State of Residence-National Vital Statistics System, United States, 2012(2014). Available from: https://www.cdc.gov/mmwr/preview/mmwrhtml/mm6320a6.htm.
3. March of Dimes (MOD). Born too soon: the global action report on preterm birth. 2015. Available from: https://www.marchofdimes.org/mission/global-preterm.aspx.
4. Brown HK, Speechley KN, Macnab J, Natale R, Campbell MK. Neonatal morbidity associated with late preterm and early term birth: the roles of gestational age and biological determinants of preterm birth. Int J Epidemiol. 2014;43(3):802–14. https://doi.org/10.1093/ije/dyt251. Epub. PubMed PMID: 24374829; PubMed Central PMCID: PMC4052131.
5. World Bank. Report on Malawi. Washington, DC: The World Bank Group; 2013.
6. World Health Organization (WHO). The WHO African Health observatory. (2015). Available from: http://www.aho.afro.who.int/profiles_information/index.php/Malawi:Analytical_summary_-_Service_delivery.
7. World Health Organization (WHO). WHO recommendations on interventions to improve preterm birth outcomes. Geneva: World Health Organization; 2015.
8. Chan GJ, Valsangkar B, Kajeepeta S, Boundy EO, Wall S. What is kangaroo mother care? Systematic review of the literature. J Glob Health. 2016;6(1):010701. Available from: https://www.ncbi.nlm.nih.gov/pubmed/27231546.
9. World Health Organization (WHO). World health statistics – 2014. Geneva: World Health Organization; 2014. Available from: https://knoema.com/UNWHODATA2014/un-world-health-statistics-2014?location=1001930-zambia&variable=1002040-preterm-birth-rate-per-100-live-births.

10. UNICEF. Maternal and Newborn Health Disparities Zambia. New York: UNICEF; 2015.
11. Macado AKF, Marmitt LP, Cesar JA. Late preterm birth in the far south of Brazil: a population based study. Rev Bras Saude Matern Infant. 2016;16(2). Available from: http://www.scielo.br/scielo.php?script=sci_arttext&pid=S1519-38292016000200113.
12. Save the Children. Time to focus on 84 000 preterm births in South Africa. Sango Pulse Net. 2012. Available from: http://www.ngopulse.org/press-release/time-focus-84-000-preterm-births-south-africa.

The Alternative Facts About Late Preterm Infants: You Mean There Are Fake Stories About Me?

Shahirose Sadrudin Premji, Gisela Becker, Katherine Bright, Genevieve Currie, Aliyah Dosani, Susan Kau, Carole Kenner, Karen Lasby, Mary R. Landsiedel, Abhay K. Lodha, Jennifer Marandola, Lenora Marcellus, Allison C. Munn, Gianella Santos Pana, Catherine Ringham, and Sarah N. Taylor

S. S. Premji (✉)
School of Nursing, Faculty of Health, York University, Toronto, ON, Canada
e-mail: premjis@yorku.ca

G. Becker
Department of Health and Community Services, Government of Newfoundland and Labrador, St. John's, NL, Canada
e-mail: GiselaBecker@gov.nl.ca

K. Bright
Faculty of Nursing, University of Calgary, Calgary, AB, Canada

Women's Mental Health Clinic, Alberta Health Services, Calgary, AB, Canada
e-mail: ksbright@ucalgary.ca; Katherine.Bright@albertahealthservices.ca

G. Currie
School of Nursing and Midwifery, Mount Royal University, Calgary, AB, Canada
e-mail: Gcurrie@mtroyal.ca

A. Dosani
School of Nursing and Midwifery, Mount Royal University, Calgary, AB, Canada
e-mail: adosani@mtroyal.ca

S. Kau
Caring for Hawai'i Neonates, Honolulu, HI, USA

Council of International Neonatal Nurses, Inc. (COINN), Yardley, PA, USA

C. Kenner
School of Nursing and Health and Exercise Science, The College of New Jersey, New York, NY, USA

Council of International Neonatal Nurses, Inc. (COINN), Yardley, PA, USA

K. Lasby
Neonatal Transition Team, Postpartum Services, Calgary, AB, Canada
e-mail: karen.lasby@albertahealthservices.ca

© Springer International Publishing AG, part of Springer Nature 2019
S. S. Premji (ed.), *Late Preterm Infants*, https://doi.org/10.1007/978-3-319-94352-7_11

M. R. Landsiedel
Bachelor of Midwifery Program, School of Nursing and Midwifery, Mount Royal University,
Calgary, AB, Canada
e-mail: mlandsiedel@mtroyal.ca

A. K. Lodha
Department of Paediatrics, Cumming School of Medicine, University of Calgary,
Calgary, AB, Canada

Department of Community Health Sciences, Cumming School of Medicine, University of
Calgary, Calgary, AB, Canada

Department of Paeditrics, Foothills Medical Center C211, Alberta Health Services, Calgary,
AB, Canada

J. Marandola
volet Jeunesse/Santé-Publique, Centre intégré universitaire de santé et de services
sociaux de l'Ouest-de-l'île-de-Montréal, Montréal, QC, Canada

L. Marcellus
School of Nursing, University of Victoria, Victoria, BC, Canada

A. C. Munn
Department of Nursing, Francis Marion University, Florence, SC, USA

G. S. Pana
Birth Doula, Chavah Childbirth Services Inc., Calgary, AB, Canada

Faculty of Nursing, University of Calgary, Calgary, AB, Canada
e-mail: gspana@ucalgary.ca

C. Ringham
Faculty of Health, University of Calgary, Calgary, AB, Canada
e-mail: clringha@ucalgary.ca

S. N. Taylor
Department of Pediatrics, Medical University of South Carolina, Charleston, SC, USA
e-mail: Taylorse@musc.edu

11.1 Introduction

Late preterm infant (LPI) is a terminology that reflects our understanding that these babies are born at a critical time when the brain, lungs, and other body organs are still growing and developing [1]. We have attempted to share the growing body of evidence that provide insight into the characteristics of these infants that threaten their adaptation outside the uterus (i.e., womb), present as challenges to health-care providers and parents, and impact growth and neurodevelopmental outcomes of LPIs. LPIs have taught us much along the way; however, work place organization (e.g., technology, policies, procedures) creates competing demands in skillfully caring for LPI. We find that LPIs are sometimes treated as normal infants leaving parents with an impression that these babies are not a "big deal" ([2], p. 1). The myths (i.e., false beliefs or ideas) that frame our (health-care providers, parents, and families) perspective about LPIs create difficulties in being responsive to LPIs and hinder our ability to care for LPIs in ways that will enable them to reach their full potential. In this final chapter, we share misconceptions about LPIs and their families and provide facts that will provide pause to rethink your approach to care.

Myth #1: The management of late preterm labor including moving to delivery as the infant is "almost term" and should be "doing well."

Fact: Recent evidence suggests that expectant management may be more appropriate during the late preterm phase resulting in improved neonatal outcomes. This involves careful monitoring by health-care professionals including continuous surveillance if rupture of membranes has occurred and occasionally a hospital admission.

Myth #2: I'm a normal healthy baby.

Fact: Late preterm infants (LPIs) arrive 4–6 weeks early, and they are masterpieces in the making, especially their brain architect and function. Address their challenges related to jaundice, feeding, hypothermia, etc., in a timely way so it does not impact the development of their brain.

Myth #3: LPIs are at no greater risk to develop hypoglycemia than term infants.

Fact: Late preterm infants show signs of hypoglycemia at a rate three times higher than term newborns; they have limited glycogen stores and immature liver function. Make sure that you anticipate hypoglycemia in LPIs, communicate with the most responsible provider, and follow current and evidence-based protocols for successful treatment without unnecessarily disrupting the mother-infant relationship.

Myth #4: Mothers of LPIs are at no greater risk for emotional health concerns than mothers of term infants.

Fact: The preterm birth impairs the mother's opinion of her ability to "mother" her newborn, and the uncertainty of the early days adds to emotional distress of women with LPI. As a result, these women experience an increase in symptoms of anxiety, depression, and post-traumatic stress disorder (PTSD). The immature brains of LPIs further contribute to maternal difficulties in responding, interacting, bonding, and attaching and significantly impact maternal sensitivity and maternal-infant attachment. Please exhibit compassion to these women, they would benefit not only from you showing empathy but also from you actively helping them during this difficult time.

Myth #5: Fathers do not influence neurodevelopment of preterm infants including LPIs.

Fact: Two-sided vocalizations or conversations during paternal-infant interactions promote communication and language development later in life (1–3 years of age). Emerging evidence suggests that fathers of LPIs may have less verbal interactions and respond less frequently to their infant's vocalization from birth through 7 months when compared to mothers. Fathers feel like they are in the periphery of maternal, newborn, and child health care since parenting is stereotypically focused on mothers. Health-care providers should make fathers feel more included and encourage parent talk to enhance paternal-infant interactions to enable LPIs to reach their full developmental potential.

Myth #6: Fathers do not contribute in the area of breastfeeding success.

Fact: Duration of skin-to-skin with fathers during the first day after birth, rather than the mother, was associated with exclusive breastfeeding at discharge. When fathers practiced skin-to-skin care with their LPIs during the first and second day of life, it was comparably less than half the time LPIs spend skin-to-skin with their mother. This indicates that there is potential opportunity to improve rates of exclusive breastfeeding through paternal caregiving environments. Health-care providers should provide ample opportunities and time for fathers to practice skin-to-skin with their LPI to improve infant health.

Myth #7: Parents of LPIs do not require any extra support.

Fact: As health professionals we need to recognize that LPIs will have ongoing issues when discharged home including risk of jaundice and difficulties with feeding which may require readmission. Anticipatory guidance will better prepare parents and may reduce their stress and self-confidence in care.

Myth #8: The plans of care for the LPI are the same.

Fact: Clinical problems—respiratory distress, apnea/bradycardia/desaturations (A/B/Ds), temperature instability, hypoglycemia, hyperbilirubinemia, and problems breast/bottle feeding—vary in presentation and duration which reinforces the need for individualized care.

Myth #9: Safe, individualized care of LPIs is assured when care providers use evidence-based guidelines, policies, and technology in their practice.

Fact: We assume that standardized technology like medication libraries, barcode systems on medications and breast milk, glucometers, and feeding pumps prevent errors and make patient care safer and more efficient. However, safety-promoting tools, like these, demand a significant portion of nurses' attention. Arduous processes connected to many technologies interfere with nurses' capacity to provide safe individualized care. Nurses must deliberately bring the infants in their care back to the center of their view and push the demands of institutional policies and technology to the periphery. The risks associated with LPIs will be mitigated with 1:1 attention *on the baby,* at critical points in their development.

Myth #10: In the neonatal intensive care unit (NICU), feeding LPIs is fun and easy work.

Fact: Within NICU contexts, nurses' feeding-related knowledge and their work with LPIs are often overlooked and underestimated in comparison to infants who are more ill. NICU nurses are acutely attuned to subtle infant feeding cues, skilled in assessment of feeding-related physiology, expert at facilitating infant-parent relationships, and able to carefully manipulate feeding equipment (bottles and nipples, gavage tubes, IV pumps) in response to infant needs. Using the criteria of 3-hourly feeding intervals and 30 minutes to feed each infant, and a typical level 1 or 2 NICU caseload of caring for 3–4 LPIs who are close to discharge, nurses invest close to two-thirds of each 12-h shift in complex feeding work. Consider the other work that NICU nurses are required to navigate in the remaining portion of their shift: medication delivery, assessment, charting, parent education and support, and so on. How are nurses supported to accomplish the complex feeding work inside many competing demands?

Myth #11: LPIs who meet the weight requirements for care by parent in the postnatal ward can be discharged within 48 h like term infants.

Fact: Despite their appearance and weight, LPIs who are discharged early more frequently require readmission to hospital. Readmission rates for the LPI are up to three times more frequent with infants discharged less than 48 h after birth more likely to be readmitted. The leading cause of readmission for the LPI is hyperbilirubinemia complicated by breastfeeding challenges leading to dehydration and weight loss. Discharge planning for the LPI that includes assessment of effective feeding, documentation of bilirubin levels, parental readiness to care for the LPI, and detailed follow-up in the community including a visit in 24–48 with lactation support can help prevent readmission. To optimize successful transition home, community care should include health-care professionals who understand the unique challenges LPIs and their families face.

Myth #12: All bottles and nipples rated for newborns have a standard flow rate.

Fact: There is no industry standard as to what constitutes a "newborn" flow rate. In fact, there is considerable variability in flow rates of newborn nipples; the rate can vary from 6 mL/min (the slowest flow nipple available) to in excess of 60 mL/min! Nipple choice will impact the LPI's suck-swallow-breathe coordination. If the nipple is too fast for the LPI's suck-swallow-breathe skill, the baby will demonstrate "flooding": squirming or restlessness while sucking, spilling while sucking, facial expression of surprise or panic (blinking, bulging eyes, and raised eyebrows), coughing, choking, or arching. Babies should exhibit relaxed body and face while sucking from a bottle. Parents should be taught signs of flooding that indicates the flow rate is inappropriate or unsafe for their LPI. Transition of LPIs to a commercial nipple before hospital discharge facilitates safe, effective, and pleasurable feedings for babies and parents.

Myth #13: A breastfeeding LPI is adequately emptying the breast.

Fact: Even if a breastfeeding LPI is taking an adequate supply of milk to remain hydrated and maintain normal level of glucose in the blood, he/she may not be removing adequate milk to stimulate appropriate increase in milk supply. Breast pumping or hand expression should be performed after direct breastfeeding during at least the first postnatal days to ensure establishment of milk supply.

Myth #14: All LPIs require supplementation and will never be able to exclusively breastfeed.

Fact: While most LPIs will require short-term supplementation during the first few months, this can vary per infant and should be assessed at each feed. It is important that parents are taught to pay attention to hunger and disengagement cues to assess whether their infant needs to be fed. Supplementation needs should take into account the size of the infant's stomach, the efficacy of the feed at the breast, and discussions with the parents. Doing so will help the parents meet the short-term needs of the infant as well as lay the groundwork for being able to eventually wean their infant off of supplementation when it is no longer necessary.

Myth #15: LPIs maintain adequate suction pressure to feed efficiently.

Fact: LPIs who latch well initially often lack the strength to maintain effective suction pressure for the duration of feedings. Mothers may offer non-nutritive sucking and tactile and sensory stimulation to prepare the infant for feedings. However, growth and oral feeding experiences are essential for developing the required strength and skill to transfer mothers' milk effectively. Parents may need to use supplemental feeding strategies until their LPI can maintain adequate suction pressure. Additionally, mothers may utilize a breast pump to promote milk supply until the infant matures and can adequately empty the breast. [Allison]

Myth #16: LPIs can consistently coordinate suck, swallow, and breathing patterns during feeding.

Fact: LPIs lack the physical maturity and often demonstrate inconsistent coordination of the suck, swallow, and breathing pathway during and between feedings. Compromised feeding coordination presents as signs of infant stress and disorganization (i.e., turning away from the breast or bottle, color changes while feeding, and pooling of milk from the mouth) and may lead to choking and regurgitation. Parents should feed when the infant is alert and interested and use cue-based feedings as this decreases infant stress, aids in suck-swallow-breathe coordination, and promotes successful feedings. Parents can provide a feeding environment that enhances infant self-regulation (e.g., encourage pauses between infant sucks) and use feeding positions that provide postural support that is adaptive to infant feeding.

Myth #17: LPIs look like term infants on the outside so their brains must also function like term infants.

Fact: LPIs are born with smaller brains than term infants. They require special attention in the early months to ensure that the brain is developing appropriately. Because of their incomplete brain development at birth, LPIs may experience developmental delay in the form of behavior, speech, and learning disorders. It is vital that parents and caregivers pay special attention to the cues LPIs give and respond appropriately. To promote healthy development, LPIs may require individualized care that includes follow-up with a multidisciplinary team to ensure that developmental milestones are met.

Myth #18: LPIs' brain development has no impact on other body systems.

Fact: Brain development does influence other body systems. For example, brain development is largely responsible for the coordination of feeding and breathing behaviors. The ability of LPIs to coordinate eating and breathing reflects the level of maturation of various structures and pathways in the brain. Therefore, parents and caregivers must pay attention to the feeding and breathing cues that LPIs are giving and respond in meaningful ways, to promote neuronal connectivity in the brain.

References

1. Kugelman A, Colin AA. Late preterm infants: near term but still in a critical developmental time period. Pediatrics. 2013;132(4):741–51. https://doi.org/10.1542/peds.2013-1131.
2. Premji SS, Currie G, Reilly S, Dosani A, Oliver LM, Lodha AK, Young M. A qualitative study: mothers of late preterm infants relate their experiences of community-based care. PLoS One. 2017;12(3):e0174419. https://doi.org/10.1371/journal.pone.0174419.